T0253827

Lecture Notes in Computer Science   8908

Commenced Publication in 1973
Founding and Former Series Editors:
Gerhard Goos, Juris Hartmanis, and Jan van Leeuwen

More information about this series at http://www.springer.com/series/7409

Hugo Plácido da Silva · Andreas Holzinger
Stephen Fairclough · Dennis Majoe (Eds.)

Physiological Computing Systems

First International Conference, PhyCS 2014
Lisbon, Portugal, January 7–9, 2014
Revised Selected Papers

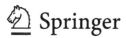 Springer

Editors

Hugo Plácido da Silva
IT - Instituto de Telecomunicações
Lisbon
Portugal

Stephen Fairclough
Liverpool John Moores
Liverpool, Merseyside
UK

Andreas Holzinger
Medical University Graz
Graz
Austria

Dennis Majoe
ETH Zurich
Zurich
Switzerland

ISSN 0302-9743   ISSN 1611-3349 (electronic)
Lecture Notes in Computer Science
ISBN 978-3-662-45685-9   ISBN 978-3-662-45686-6 (eBook)
DOI 10.1007/978-3-662-45686-6

Library of Congress Control Number: 2014957647

LNCS Sublibrary: SL3 – Information Systems and Applications, incl. Internet/Web, and HCI

Printed on acid-free paper

Springer-Verlag GmbH Berlin Heidelberg is part of Springer Science+Business Media
(www.springer.com)

Preface

The International Conference on Physiological Computing Systems (PhyCS 2014) was held in Lisbon, Portugal, during January 7–9, 2014, with the organization and sponsorship of the Institute for Systems and Technologies of Information, Control, and Communication (INSTICC).

This was the first in a series of annual meetings of the physiological interaction and computing community, and serves as the main international forum for engineers, computer scientists, and health professionals, interested in outstanding research and development that bridges the gap between physiological data handling and human-computer interaction. In 2014, PhyCS had the cooperation of the ACM SIGCHI, FP7 EMOTE, FP7 CuPiD, and FP7 ABC and also had the support and collaboration of Philips Research, Carnegie Mellon | Portugal, MIT | Portugal, Fraunhofer AICOS, and several other partners.

Physiological data in its different dimensions, either bioelectrical, biomechanical, biochemical, or biophysical, and collected through specialized biomedical devices, video and image capture, or other sources, is opening new boundaries in the field of human-computer interaction into what can be defined as Physiological Computing. Given the topical nature of this subject, PhyCS 2014 brought together people interested in creating novel interaction devices, adaptable interfaces, algorithms, and tools, through the study, planning, and design of interfaces between people and computers that are supported by multimodal biosignals. Researchers attending PhyCS sought to extend the state of the art by harnessing the power of physiological data to refine the symbiosis between humans and computers in such a way that the resulting interactive experiences lead to richer and improved outcomes.

Papers accepted in the event related to synergetic disciplines such as biomedical engineering, computer science, electrical engineering, affective computing, accessibility, usability, computer graphics, arts, etc., and addressed topics such as the design of new wearable devices that make physiological data acquisition more pervasive, the design of user interfaces capable of recognizing and adapting to changes in the physiological state of the user, and/or the creation of algorithms to enable robust and seamless control of computational resources using physiological data sources as input.

The conference received 52 submissions of which only 13 papers have been accepted as full papers. This volume is a collection of the best 10 papers, resulting in a final acceptance rate of approximately 20 %. We would like to express our gratitude, first of all, to the contributing authors of the technical papers, whose work and dedication made it possible to put together an exciting program of high technical quality. We would also like to thank all the members of the international Program Committee and auxiliary reviewers, who provided a comprehensive set of thoughtful reviews, helping us with their expertise and time. We would also like to thank the invited speakers for their invaluable contribution and for sharing their vision in their talks. We are especially grateful to the INSTICC Steering Committee whose invaluable work made this event possible.

October 2014

Hugo Plácido da Silva
Andreas Holzinger
Stephen Fairclough
Dennis Majoe

Organization

Conference Chair

Hugo Plácido da Silva   IT - Instituto de Telecomunicações, Portugal

Program Co-chairs

Andreas Holzinger   Medical University of Graz, Austria
Stephen Fairclough   Liverpool John Moores University, UK
Dennis Majoe   ETH Zurich, Switzerland

Industrial Co-chairs

Chad Stephens   NASA Langley Research Center, USA
Oliver Brdiczka   XEROX Palo Alto Research Center, USA
Jakub Tkaczuk   Samsung R&D Institute, Poland

Program Committee

Julio Abascal   University of the Basque Country, Spain
Jean-Marie Aerts   M3-BIORES, Katholieke Universitëit Leuven,
           Belgium
Jesús Alonso   Universidad de Las Palmas de Gran Canaria, Spain
Philip Azariadis   University of the Aegean, Greece
Panagiotis D. Bamidis   Aristotle University of Thessaloniki, Greece
Bert-Jan van Beijnum   University of Twente, The Netherlands
Juan-Manuel Belda-Lois   Instituto de Biomecánica de València, Spain
Sergi Bermudez i Badia   Madeira Interactive Technologies Institute/
           Universidade da Madeira, Portugal
Bir Bhanu   University of California, Riverside, USA
Dinesh Bhatia   Deenbandhu Chhotu Ram University of Science
           and Technology, India
Luciano Boquete   University of Alcalá, Spain
Jovan Brankov   Illinois Institute of Technology, USA
Ahmet Çakir   ERGONOMIC Institute, Germany
Mónica Cameirão   Madeira Interactive Technologies Institute,
           Portugal
Tolga Can   Middle East Technical University, Turkey
M. Emre Celebi   Louisiana State University in Shreveport, USA
Guillaume Chanel   University of Geneva, Switzerland
Wei Cheng   Garena Online Pte. Ltd., Singapore

Pietro Cipresso	IRCCS Istituto Auxologico Italiano, Italy
Miguel Coimbra	Faculdade de Ciências da Universidade do Porto, Portugal
Diane Cook	Washington State University, USA
David Cornforth	University of Newcastle, Australia
Fernando Cruz	Escola Superior de Tecnologia de Setúbal – IPS, Portugal
Antoine Danchin	AMAbiotics SAS, France
Thomas Dandekar	University of Würzburg, Germany
Farzin Deravi	University of Kent, UK
Sérgio Deusdado	Instituto Politecnico de Bragança, Portugal
Gintautas Dzemyda	Vilnius University, Lithuania
George Eleftherakis	International Faculty of the University of Sheffield, Greece
Mireya Fernández Chimeno	Universitat Politècnica de Catalunya, Spain
Leonardo Franco	Universidad de Málaga, Spain
Claude Frasson	University of Montreal, Canada
Christoph Friedrich	University of Applied Science and Arts Dortmund, Germany
André Gagalowicz	Inria, France
Juan Carlos Garcia Garcia	Universidad de Alcalá, Spain
Max Garzon	University of Memphis, USA
Kiel Gilleade	Liverpool John Moores University, UK
Daniel Gonçalves	INESC-id/Instituto Superior Técnico, Portugal
David Greenhalgh	University of Strathclyde, UK
Tiago Guerreiro	University of Lisbon, Portugal
Leontios Hadjileontiadis	Aristotle University of Thessaloniki, Greece
Andras Hajdu	University of Debrecen, Hungary
Andrew Hamilton-Wright	Mount Allison University, Canada
Thomas Hinze	Friedrich Schiller University Jena, Germany
Eivind Hovig	Norwegian Radium Hospital, Norway
Hailiang Huang	Massachusetts General Hospital, USA
Joris Janssen	Philips Research Europe, The Netherlands
Bo Jin	Sigma-Aldrich, USA
Sergi Jorda	Pompeu Fabra University, Spain
Joaquim Jorge	INESC-id/Instituto Superior Técnico, Portugal
Ricardo Jota	University of Toronto, Canada
Anastasia Kastania	Athens University of Economics and Business, Greece
Jonghwa Kim	University of Augsburg, Germany
Stefanos Kollias	National Technical University of Athens, Greece
Shin'ichi Konomi	University of Tokyo, Japan
Dimitri Konstantas	University of Geneva, Switzerland
Georgios Kontaxakis	Universidad Politécnica de Madrid, Spain

Egon van den Broek	University of Twente/Radboud UMC Nijmegen, The Netherlands
Iolanda Leite	INESC-id/Instituto Superior Técnico, Portugal
Hongen Liao	Tsinghua University, China
Chun-Cheng Lin	National Chiao Tung University, Taiwan
Huei-Yung Lin	National Chung Cheng University, Taiwan
Giuseppe Liotta	University of Perugia, Italy
Paulo Lobato Correia	Instituto Superior Técnico, Portugal
Martin Lopez-Nores	University of Vigo, Spain
Mai Mabrouk	Misr University for Science and Technology, Egypt
Jarmo Malinen	Aalto University, Finland
Dan Mandru	Technical University of Cluj Napoca, Romania
Francesco Marcelloni	University of Pisa, Italy
Elena Marchiori	Radboud University, The Netherlands
Jan Mares	Institute of Chemical Technology Prague, Czech Republic
Jorge Martins	Instituto Superior Técnico, Portugal
Alice Maynard	Future Inclusion, UK
Gianluigi Me	Università degli Studi di Roma "Tor Vergata", Italy
Gerrit Meixner	Heilbronn University, Germany
Nuno Mendes	Instituto de Biologia Experimental e Tecnológica, Portugal
Silvano Mignanti	Sapienza University of Rome, Italy
Ji Ming	Queen's University Belfast, UK
Yehya Mohamad	Fraunhofer FIT, Germany
Pedro Tiago	Monteiro INESC-id, Portugal
Umberto Morbiducci	Politecnico di Torino, Italy
Mihaela Morega	University Politehnica of Bucharest, Romania
Alexandru Morega	University Politehnica of Bucharest, Romania
Hammadi Nait-Charif	Bournemouth University, UK
Nicoletta Nicolaou	Imperial College London, UK
Domen Novak	ETH Zurich, Switzerland
Ian Oakley	Ulsan National Institute of Science and Technology, Korea
Rui Pedro Paiva	University of Coimbra, Portugal
Gonzalo Pajares	Universidad Complutense de Madrid, Spain
Richard Pak	Clemson University, USA
Krzysztof Pancerz	University of Information Technology and Management, Poland
Chaoyi Pang	CSIRO/The Australian e-Health Research Centre, Australia
George Panoutsos	The University of Sheffield, UK
Joao Papa	Universidade Estadual Paulista (UNESP), Brazil
José Pazos-Arias	University of Vigo, Spain
Evan Peck	Tufts University, USA

Quan Wen	University of Electronic Science and Technology of China, china
Joyce Westerink	Philips Research Europe, The Netherlands
Nicholas Wickstrom	Halmstad University, Sweden
Pew-Thian Yap	University of North Carolina at Chapel Hill, USA
Erliang Zeng	University of South Dakota, USA
Huiru Zheng	University of Ulster, UK
Leming Zhou	University of Pittsburgh, USA
Li Zhuo	Beijing University of Technology, China
André Zúquete	IEETA/IT/Universidade de Aveiro, Portugal

Organizing Committee

Bruno Encarnação	INSTICC, Portugal

Partners

We are grateful to the following companies and institutions for their support in our aims to bridge Science and Industry: ACM In-Cooperation, ACM SIGCHI, Anditec – Tecnologias de Reabilitação, Carnegie Mellon | Portugal, FP7 EMOTE, FP7 CuPiD, FP7 ABC, Fraunhofer AICOS, Fundação PT, Health Cluster Portugal, INSTICC – Institute for Systems and Technologies of Information Control and Communication, IT – Instituto de Telecomunicações, MIT | Portugal, Philips Research, PLUX – Wireless Biosignals, SAPO Labs, SCITEEVENTS, SCITEPRESS, SCITESOFT.

Contents

Human Factors

Methodologies and Methods

Wavelet Lifting over Information-Based EEG Graphs for Motor Imagery Data Classification

Javier Asensio-Cubero[1]([⊠]), John Q. Gan[1], and Ramaswamy Palaniappan[2]

[1] University of Essex, Wivenhoe Park, Colchester, Essex CO4 3SQ, UK
{jasens,jqgan}@essex.ac.uk
[2] University of Wolverhampton, Shifnal Road, Telford TF2 9NT, UK
palani@wlv.ac.uk

Abstract. The imagination of limb movements offers an intuitive paradigm for the control of electronic devices via brain computer interfacing (BCI). The analysis of electroencephalographic (EEG) data related to motor imagery potentials has proved to be a difficult task. EEG readings are noisy, and the elicited patterns occur in different parts of the scalp, at different instants and at different frequencies. Wavelet transform has been widely used in the BCI field as it offers temporal and spectral capabilities, although it lacks spatial information. In this study we propose a tailored second generation wavelet to extract features from these three domains. This transform is applied over a graph representation of motor imaginary trials, which encodes temporal and spatial information. This graph is enhanced using per-subject knowledge in order to optimise the spatial relationships among the electrodes, and to improve the filter design. This method improves the performance of classifying different imaginary limb movements maintaining the low computational resources required by the lifting transform over graphs. By using an online dataset we were able to positively assess the feasibility of using the novel method in an online BCI context.

Keywords: Multiresolution analysis · EEG data graph representation · Motor imagery · Brain computer interfacing · Wavelet lifting · Mutual information

1 Introduction

Brain signal analysis, applied for the control of computerised devices, is critical for a human-machine interaction paradigm known as brain-computer interfacing (BCI). This new way of communication not only has a direct positive impact on motor disabled users in terms of quality of life and interaction with their surroundings, but also opens new modes of operation for healthy users to interact with their environment.

The human brain responds to different stimuli with alterations in its neural activity. These alterations, which manifest as changes in the electrical activity in the cortex and changing blood oxygen levels in different regions, can

© Springer-Verlag Berlin Heidelberg 2014
H.P. da Silva et al. (Eds.): PhyCS 2014, LNCS 8908, pp. 3–19, 2014.
DOI: 10.1007/978-3-662-45686-6_1

be measured with appropriate technology. In terms of electrical activity, these responses provoke oscillations known as event related potentials (ERP) that can be measured with electroencephalographic (EEG) devices and detected with appropriate algorithms [11].

One example of an ERP is from the imagination of limb movements, which is commonly known as motor imagery (MI). Depending on the limb involved, the brain activity derived from MI tasks produces changes in neural activity on different parts of the brain cortex, at different rates and with different temporal behaviour. These changes produce a series of short lasting amplifications and attenuations in the EEG data known as event related desynchronisation (ERD) and event related synchronisation (ERS) [17].

The study of ERS/ERD has proven to be a hard task. EEG data is noisy and of low amplitude, there is no inter-subject pattern consistency, and features that make the ERS/ERD patterns recognisable appear at different time intervals, different scalp locations and different frequency bands.

Wavelets have been profusely applied in the BCI domain as they allow a meaningful temporal-spectral analysis of the EEG data. Shifts and dilations of a mother wavelet function provide a series of orthogonal subspaces resulting in what is known as multi-resolution analysis (MRA) [10]. First generation wavelets present a major disadvantage of difficult design. Researchers usually make use of well established wavelet families, even though the wavelet function features may not completely fulfil the needs of the domain of study.

On the other hand, during the last decade a new wavelet framework has become popular for building tailored wavelets. Wavelet lifting, often referred to as second generation wavelets, offers a simple framework to construct wavelet functions that have fewer restrictions and can be applied in a natural way to many situations that first generation wavelets are incapable of handling [23,24].

The possibilities offered by the lifting transform open new interesting ways to look at BCI signal processing. In [1] a new MRA system for BCI data analysis was proposed using lifting scheme over graphs to fully explore the three domains involved in ERS/ERD patterns evolution. Graph EEG data representation is a natural way of describing the spatio/temporal relations among electrode readings. The purpose of this study is to extend the static graph representation by automatically building an enhanced graph in which the connections represent meaningful relationships among different electrodes. For this purpose we used mutual information as it provides a measurement of how much information one channel shares with another channel.

The paper is organised as follows: data acquisition is detailed in Sects. 2.1, 2.2 explains the lifting scheme over graphs, Sect. 2.3 describes how the graphs are built, Sect. 2.4 focuses on the feature extraction technique, pattern description and classification methods, and the experimental methodology is described in Sect. 2.5. The obtained results along with discussions are presented in Sect. 3. Finally, the conclusions are drawn in Sect. 4.

2 Methods

2.1 Data Acquisition and Preprocessing

The first dataset was recorded at the BCI Laboratory at the University of Essex. The protocol was set up as follows: The electrode placement followed the 10–20 international system and 32 channels were recorded with a sampling frequency of 256 Hz. During the recording session the subject was sitting on an arm-chair in front of a computer screen. A fixation cross was showed at the beginning of the trial at $t = 0$ s. At $t = 2$ s a cue was shown indicating the imaginary movement class to perform. The end of the trial was marked when the fixation cross and cue disappeared at $t = 8$ s. The subjects were asked to perform 120 trials from each of the three imaginary movements (right hand, left hand and feet). A total of 12 subjects participated in the recording sessions, half of them were naive on the use of BCI systems, 58 % of the subjects were female, and the ages ranged from 24 to 50. During the result analysis these subjects were identified by the prefix E-X, with X being the subject number.

The second dataset is from the BCI Competition IV (dataset 2a) and follows a similar acquisition protocol. The full experiment description can be found in [5]. The data consists of four different types of MI movements: right-hand, left-hand, feet and tongue. For each of the nine subjects a total of 288 trials recorded with a sampling frequency of 250 Hz. The subjects belonging to this dataset are identified by the prefix C-X.

The calibration trials in the third dataset were acquired following an identical protocol of the first dataset. The validation trials were recorded while the subject controlled a BCI system in real-time with continuous feedback. The results for the online classification were not the ones described here, since the data was reprocessed offline for this study. Twelve healthy subjects took part in the experiment, all of whom were naive to the use of online BCI. The subjects were aged from 24 to 32 and 50 % were female. The subjects in this dataset are labeled with the prefix O-X.

For this study we utilised a subset of 15 electrodes, covering the major area of the motor cortex (Fig. 1). The original data was filtered from 8 to 30 Hz in order to attenuate external noise and artifacts. Each trial X_i of T samples was scaled by applying $X_i = \frac{1}{\sqrt{T}} X_i^{orig} (I_t - 1_t 1_t')$, where I_t is the $T \times T$ identity matrix and 1_t is a T dimensional vector with ones in it.

The competition data was already divided into training and evaluation subsets. The off-line data from the University of Essex was split using the first two acquisition runs (180 trials) as training data and the last two runs (180 trials) as evaluation set. The data from the online experiment contained 160 trials for calibration and 90 trials for validation purposes.

2.2 Wavelet Lifting over EEG Graphs

First generation wavelets represent signals in terms of shifts and dilations of the basis function known as mother wavelet. The design of this function obeys a

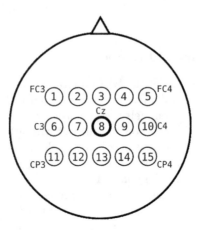

Fig. 1. Numbering of the 15 electrodes used during the experimentation, which were allocated from FC3 to FC4, C3 to C4, and CP3 to CP4.

set of restrictions assuring an accurate orthogonal decomposition of the original data. The main benefit of wavelet analysis over other orthogonal systems, such as the Fourier transform or the cosine transform, is its multiscale capability. Wavelets allow to analyse the data not only in the frequency domain, but also in the temporal domain at different levels [10, 12].

The use of first generation wavelets is pervasive in many domains where signal processing is involved, and BCIs are no exception. In P-300 based BCIs wavelet decomposition is commonly used as the method of signal analysis. In [4] non-parametric statistics from the different levels of a Mexican hat common wavelet transform were adopted. The Daubechies wavelet in its discrete variant was applied in [16] using the thresholded coefficients as feature vectors for classification.

There are also several examples of wavelet transforms used in MI-based BCIs. In [18] Morlet wavelets were used to decompose signals of imaginary limb movements. In [6] discrete wavelet transform was applied using different families (Daubechies, Coiflets and Symlets), sub-band power and the standard deviation of the analysis and detail coefficients at different levels were used as feature extraction method. In [26] Coiflet decompositions of fifth order were used, as they claimed that its shape is the closest to the ERD/ERS.

It is rarer to find the wavelet transform in the study of SSVEP BCIs but it has been applied, as in [25] where continuous Morlet wavelets were used to study the EEG data.

One major issue to cope with when working with the wavelet transform is that wavelet function design is an extremely complex task, and therefore, researchers apply common families in their studies despite the mother wavelet may not be suitable for the domain of study. The introduction of second generation wavelets, also known as wavelet lifting [22], alleviates this problem making the design of complete multiresolution systems more straight forward. The wavelet lifting is capable of handling data where Fourier analysis is not suitable (and therefore first generation wavelets either), such as unevenly sampled data, surfaces, spheres [20], trees [21] and graphs [13,14].

A lifting scheme consists of iterations of three basic operations [7]:

- **Split:** Separate the original signal x into two subsets, referred as odd (x_o) and even (x_e) elements.
- **Predict:** The error of predicting x_o in base of x_e using a *predictor operator* $\mathcal{P}$ conforms the wavelet coefficients d.
- **Update:** The coarser approximation of the original signal is calculated by combining x_e and d using an *update operator* $\mathcal{U}$.

A lifting transform over graphs can be defined as follows [14]. Let us consider a graph $G = (V, E)$ where V is the node set of size $N = N_o + N_e$ and E the edges linking those nodes. V is divided into the even and odd sets and E is represented using an adjacency matrix Adj. We rearrange V and Adj so that the odd set of nodes (a vector V_o of size $N_o \times 1$) is gathered before the even set (a vector V_e of size $N_e \times 1$), obtaining the following structure:

$$\tilde{V} = \begin{pmatrix} V_o \\ V_e \end{pmatrix}$$

$$\tilde{Adj} = \begin{pmatrix} F^{N_o \times N_o} & J^{N_o \times N_e} \\ K^{N_e \times N_o} & L^{N_e \times N_e} \end{pmatrix} \tag{1}$$

The submatrices F and L in $\tilde{Adj}$ in Eq. (1) are discarded as they link elements within the same node sets. The block matrices J and K contain only edges linking nodes from different node sets.

The lifting transform functions are defined using a weighted version of the block matrices J and K:

$$D = V_o - J^\omega \times V_e$$
$$A = V_e + K^\omega \times D \tag{2}$$

where the prediction and update functions are defined as a matrix product: $\mathcal{P} = J^\omega \times V_e$ and $\mathcal{U} = K^\omega \times D$, where J^ω and K^ω are the weighted adjacency block matrices and their actual values depend on the domain of application.

We repeat the process described in Eq. (2) in each level. In level $l + 1$ we assign the approximation coefficients A in level l to V.

2.3   Automatic EEG Graph Building and Filter Design

In [1], a static EEG data graph representation was introduced. This representation had the benefit of keeping a channel oriented structure although no extra information was used to optimise the inter-channel links. In order to stablish which channels should be connected for each subject we made use of the mutual information of every pair of channels [9, 15].

Mutual information measures the amount of information that one random variable Y contains about another random variable Z and is given by:

$$I(Y; Z) = \sum_{y \in Y} \sum_{z \in Z} p(y, z) log \frac{p(y, z)}{p(y)p(z)} \qquad (3)$$

where $p(y, z)$ is the joint probability mass function, $p(y)$ and $p(z)$ are the marginal probability mass functions.

Consider a set of MI trials $X^{T \times C}$ of T samples and C channels. In order to establish the relationships among the spatial locations we compute the mutual information $M(r, s) = I(c_r; c_s)$ for every pair of channels c_r c_s with $r \in \{1 \ldots C\}$ and $s \in \{1 \ldots C\}$. Note that the diagonal elements of M are set to zero (the mutual information of a channel with itself is ignored) and the rest of non-zero elements are normalised between zero and one.

The symmetric matrix M describes how all the channels are related to each other and this information can be used to build a specific graph representation for each subject.

Let us assume that the graph $G^x = (V^x, E^x)$ is embedding a trial X, where V^x defines the nodes and the edge set E^x is represented by a weighted adjacency matrix Adj^x:

$$Adj_{ij}^x = \begin{cases} a_{ij} & \text{If } v_i^x \text{ is connected to } v_j^x \\ 0 & \text{Otherwise} \end{cases} \qquad (4)$$

For convenience, the odd set will correspond to the elements of X at odd values of t, and the even set at even values of t. Therefore, we obtain two different node vectors v_o^x and v_e^x.

The *predict* and *update* filters are computed in terms of the matrices M and Adj^x. The following steps are carried out in order to set the adjacency matrix values:

1. Apply a threshold th to the matrix M such that $M(r, s) = 0$ if $M(r, s) < th$, so only those channels with high mutual information values will be linked, and normalise the non-zero values between zero and one.
2. Set Adj^x such that for a given channel c and instant t it will be connected to the previous $t - 1$ and following $t + 1$ time instants with a weight $a_{ij} = 1$.
3. For all the other channels c_r and adjacent temporal values $t + 1$ and $t - 1$ set the weight $a_{ij} = M(c, c_r)$ in the corresponding entry of Adj^x, if $M(c, c_r) > 0$.

The resulting adjacency submatrices of F^x and L^x from Adj^x are empty. The *predict* and *update* matrices $J^{\omega x}$ and $K^{\omega x}$ (weighted versions the submatrices J^x and K^x) are computed row-wise as $J_{ij}^{\omega x} = \frac{J_{ij}^x}{\sum_{k=0}^{J} J_{ik}^x}$ and $K_{ij}^{\omega x} = \frac{J_{ij}^x}{2 * \sum_{k=0}^{J} J_{ik}^x}$. It is noteworthy to mention that the obtained lifting filters are weighted Laplacian graph filters, and the design explained here ensures that those channels that share high mutual information will contribute more to the detail coefficients than those that share low mutual information.

2.4   Feature Extraction and Classification

One of the main drawbacks in the use of multiresolution analysis for signal classification is the large number of coefficients generated during the transform. In order to overcome this problem we use common spatial patterns (CSP) as a method for feature extraction and dimensionality reduction. CSP is an extension to PCA where two different classes of data are taken into account.

Assuming that the trials contains data from class (+) and class (-), a set of samples X is divided into $X^{(+)}$ and $X^{(-)}$. Their simultaneously estimated covariance matrix decomposition is given by [3]:

$$\Sigma^{(+)} = W\Lambda^{(+)}W^T$$
$$\Sigma^{(-)} = W\Lambda^{(-)}W^T \tag{5}$$

where $\Sigma^{(+)}$ is the estimated covariance matrix for the trials belonging to class (+) and $\Sigma^{(-)}$ is the covariance matrix for the trials belonging to class (-). $\Lambda^{(+)}$ and $\Lambda^{(-)}$ are diagonal matrices with the eigenvalues corresponding to the decomposition of $\Sigma^{(+)}$ and $\Sigma^{(-)}$. A large eigenvalue $\Lambda^{(+)}_{jj}$ means that the corresponding eigenvector from matrix W, $\mathbf{w}_j$, leads to high variance in the projected signal in the positive class and low variance in the negative one (and vice-versa). The CSP projection results in $Y_i = W^T X_i$.

The detail D^l and approximation A^l sets at different levels from the MRA were projected onto their own CSP subspaces $Y^{D_l} = W^T_{D_l} \times D^l$ and $Y^{A_l} = W^T_{A_l} \times A^l$. For clarity, we will refer to Y^{D_l} and Y^{A_l} using $\bar{Y}$.

For every $\bar{Y}$, we extracted the rows which maximised and minimised the variance between the two different classes (namely, the first m rows and last m rows) and calculated every feature as $f_k = var(\bar{\mathbf{y}}_k)$ with $k = \{1, 2, \ldots, m, C - (m-1), \ldots, C\}$, obtaining a total of $F = 2 * m$ features. In order to scale down the difference among the feature values, the logarithm $f_k^{log} = log(\frac{f_k}{\sum_{j=1}^F f_j})$ was computed [19].

For this study, $m \in \{2, 3, 4\}$ was chosen using cross validation as explained in Sect. 2.5.

The features obtained from the CSP were classified using LDA as it provides a fair compromise between resource consumption and classification performance [2].

In order to measure the classification performance Kappa value [8] was used instead of the classification ratio. Kappa value gives an accurate description of the classifier's performance, taking into account the per class error distribution. The Kappa value was computed as $\kappa = \frac{p_o - p_c}{1 - p_c}$, where p_o is the proportion of units on which the judgement agrees (based on the output from the classifier and the actual label), and p_c is the proportion of units on which the agreement is expected by chance.

2.5   Experimental Methodology

After the data preprocessing, a temporal sliding window of one second with a fifth of second overlap was applied over each trial. The segmented data was then transformed using a lifting scheme over graphs (See Sects. 2.2 and 2.3) to the sixth level. The transformation resulted in twelve different coefficient sets, which were further processed to obtain the feature sets by selecting different number of CSP features (See Sect. 2.4).

The MRA approaches used for comparison were:

- Graph lifting scheme with static graphs [1]. The static graph is built by linking the elements from the surrounding channels as shown in Fig. 2. The filters are calculated analogously as explained in Sect. 2.3 but by setting the weights of the Laplacian filters to one.
- Graph lifting scheme and mutual information driven graph building.

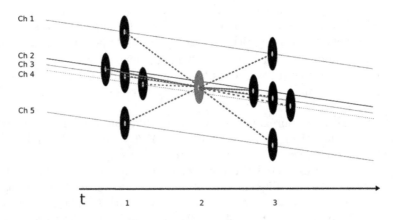

Fig. 2. Detail of the graph after the even/odd split for the static approach. The even element (in red) is linked to the surrounding odd elements (in black) adding spatial information to the decomposition (color figure online).

Each detail and approximation coefficient sets from different temporal segments were classified with a separate LDA model after applying CSP. This led to a total of $n_s * l * 2$ LDA outputs, with n_s being the number of segments and l the number of levels. A majority voting approach was carried out in order to obtain the final classification output for each trial.

A cross-validation step using five folds was performed over the training data in order to select the two free parameters involved: the threshold applied to the mutual information matrix in Sect. 2.3 and the number of CSP features as explained in Sect. 2.4.

3   Results and Discussion

From the analysis of the mutual information matrix M for the different subjects we learnt that, in general, the standard deviations of the paired calculation do not differ much when compared among classes (two orders of magnitude smaller than the mean). Therefore, instead of computing a matrix M and a different graph to process one class against the others, we just used the whole set of data to generate the mutual information based adjacency matrix. This simplifies the model decreasing the execution time. It is also noteworthy that the performance of the transform calculation does not vary although the values of the filters applied changed.

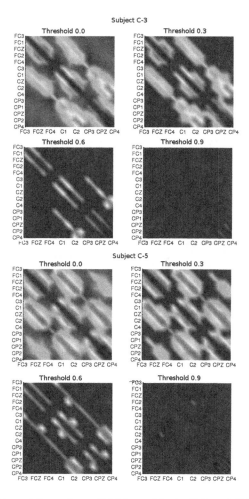

Fig. 3. Representation of the values of M for subjects C-3 and C-5 applying different thresholds

Figures 3, 4, and 5 are graphical representations of the values of the matrix M for different users and with different thresholds. In Fig. 3 we find two examples to show that there exists a clear correlation between the electrode spatial location

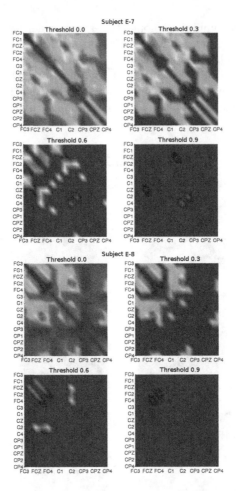

Fig. 4. Representation of the values of matrix M for subjects E-7 and E-8 applying different thresholds

and the mutual information. The parallel lines crossing the figure diagonally corresponds to high mutual information values between adjacent electrodes. This correlation is more evident if we compare it with Fig. 6, which corresponds to the matrix M of the static approach. Although in Figs. 4 to 5 this effect is still noticeable. It is more obvious how, for some specific subjects, the inter-electrode information is more prominent in particular locations of the motor cortex, concretely, in the frontal and central lobes for subject E-7 and O-2, eminently central for subject E-8, and more scattered for subject O-7.

After applying the experimental methodology described in Sect. 2.5 we can analyse the impact of the automatic graph building on the classification results. Figures 7, 8 and 9 show how the median Kappa values change when different threshold values are applied. It is clear that the behaviour of the method is dependant on the subject of analysis. Some subjects, such as E-8, C-4 and C-2,

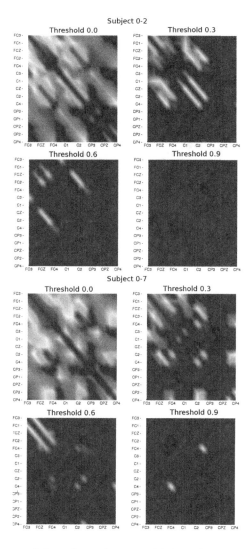

Fig. 5. Representation of the values of matrix M for subjects O-2 and O-7 applying different thresholds

are not significantly affected by the change of the threshold value, although, on the other hand, we find subjects where the Kappa value fluctuates around 0.1 depending on the threshold value such as in subjects C-3, C-7, E-9, E-11, O-1 and O-4.

After selecting the two parameters, the mutual information threshold and the number of features used in CSP, from the cross-validation results we can compute the classification performance on the evaluation data. Table 1 shows the Kappa values and mean accuracy for the Essex dataset, Table 2 for the competition dataset, and Table 3 for the online dataset.

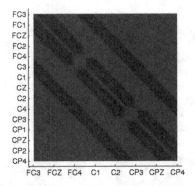

Fig. 6. Values of the matrix M for the static graph approach.

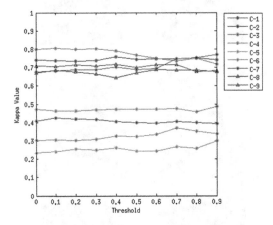

Fig. 7. Median of the Kappa value in function of the threshold applied to the matrix M for the competition dataset

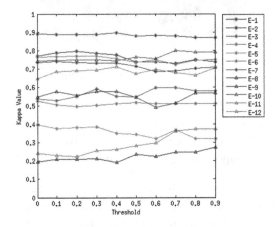

Fig. 8. Median of the Kappa value in function of the threshold applied to the matrix M for the Essex dataset

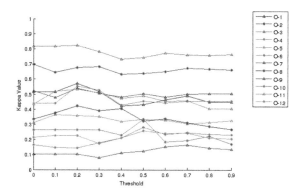

Fig. 9. Median of the Kappa value in function of the threshold applied to the matrix M for the online dataset

Table 1. Results on the Essex dataset in terms of Kappa values. The mean accuracy is included at the bottom.

Subject	GLS	GLS + Mutual Information
E-1	**0.757**	0.741
E-2	0.736	**0.744**
E-3	0.539	**0.644**
E-4	**0.730**	0.712
E-5	0.392	**0.393**
E-6	**0.529**	0.488
E-7	0.883	**0.891**
E-8	0.210	**0.263**
E-9	0.565	**0.581**
E-10	0.757	**0.774**
E-11	0.237	**0.321**
E-12	0.648	**0.707**
Mean Kappa	0.582	0.605
	±	±
	0.21	0.19
Mean Acc	0.723	0.737
	±	±
	0.14	0.13

For 78.8 % of the 33 subjects in the three datasets the proposed method achieved a higher Kappa value. For some of the subjects this improvement rises the Kappa value by 0.1 when compared to the static approach.

Table 2. Results on the competition dataset in terms of Kappa values. The mean accuracy is included at the bottom.

Subject	GLS	GLS + Mutual Information
C-1	0.754	**0.763**
C-2	0.410	**0.419**
C-3	0.800	**0.805**
C-4	0.484	0.475
C-5	0.243	**0.257**
C-6	0.317	**0.364**
C-7	0.629	**0.758**
C-8	0.661	**0.707**
C-9	0.698	**0.721**
Mean Kappa	0.555	0.586
	±	±
	0.19	0.20
Mean Acc	0.666	0.689
	±	±
	0.15	0.15

Table 3. Results on the online dataset in terms of Kappa values. The mean accuracy is included at the bottom.

Subject	GLS	GLS + Mutual Information
O-1	**0.494**	0.454
O-2	0.640	**0.711**
O-3	0.777	**0.789**
O-4	0.432	**0.541**
O-5	0.334	**0.376**
O-6	**0.306**	0.278
O-7	0.107	**0.165**
O-8	0.248	**0.376**
O-9	**0.534**	0.504
O-10	0.222	**0.320**
O-11	0.434	**0.532**
O-12	0.179	**0.263**
Mean Kappa	0.392	0.443
	±	±
	0.18	0.17
Mean Acc	0.59	0.629
	±	±
	0.12	0.11

There exists a difference between the Essex and the online datasets in terms of classification accuracy, even though the acquisition protocol was practically identical. This decrement in the classification performance is probably due to the stress suffered by the subjects during the online experiments.

As a final remark we can mention that the proposed method obtains a Kappa value of 0.586 using the competition dataset, while the winner of the competition achieved 0.57. The small number of subjects in the competition data does not allow us to carry out a definitive significance test to compare both approaches.

4 Conclusions

In this study we have proposed a novel method to improve the EEG data representation based on static graphs by using the mutual information among the different channels, which constitutes an example of the possibilities offered by second generation wavelets in the BCI domain. This new strategy for building the graph also has an impact on the filter design, allowing an automatic way to weight the contribution of the different spatial locations.

After applying the proposed methodology on the three datasets, the resulting Kappa value was increased for 78.8 % percent of the subjects obtaining for several subjects an improvement of 0.1.

From the results achieved on the online dataset we can state that the proposed method is suitable for online BCI systems, although the calibration time needed to obtain competitive results is relatively high, as the number of features used by CSP and the threshold have to be set via cross-validation.

Comparing the mutual information matrices from different subjects we can observe how the initial static graph approach, where the surrounding electrodes were linked together, was appropriate as close electrodes tend to share similar information.

These positive results encourage us to explore new ways for optimising the graph representation of EEG data. Although mutual information has helped to improve the classification rate, other techniques such as Granger causality, which could be more robust when coping with non-stationarity, should be examined in future work.

Acknowledgements. The first author would like to thank the EPSRC for funding his Ph.D. study via an EPSRC DTA award.

References

1. Asensio-Cubero, J., Gan, J.Q., Palaniappan, R.: Multiresolution analysis over simple graphs for brain computer interfaces. J. Neural Eng. **10**(4), 046014 (2013)
2. Blankertz, B., Muller, K.R., Krusienski, D.J., Schalk, G., Wolpaw, J.R., Schlogl, A., Pfurtscheller, G., Millan, J.R., Schroder, M., Birbaumer, N.: The BCI competition III: validating alternative approaches to actual BCI problems. IEEE Trans. Neural Syst. Rehabil. Eng. **14**(2), 153–159 (2006)

3. Blankertz, B., Tomioka, R., Lemm, S., Kawanabe, M., Muller, K.R.: Optimizing spatial filters for robust EEG single-trial analysis. IEEE Signal Process. Mag. **25**(1), 41–56 (2008)
4. Bostanov, V.: BCI competition 2003-data sets ib and IIb: feature extraction from event-related brain potentials with the continuous wavelet transform and the t-value scalogram. IEEE Trans. Biomed. Eng. **51**(6), 1057–1061 (2004)
5. Brunner, C., Leeb, R., Muller-Putz, G.R., Schlogl, A., Pfurtscheller, G.: BCI competition 2008 - Graz data set A (2008). http://www.bbci.de/competition/iv/desc_2a.pdf
6. Carrera-Leon, O., Ramirez, J.M., Alarcon-Aquino, V., Baker, M., D'Croz-Baron, D., Gomez-Gil, P.: A motor imagery BCI experiment using wavelet analysis and spatial patterns feature extraction. In: 2012 Workshop on Engineering Applications (WEA), pp. 1–6 (2012)
7. Claypoole Jr., R.L., Baraniuk, R.G., Nowak, R.D.: Adaptive wavelet transforms via lifting. Proceedings of IEEE International Conference on Acoustics, Speech and Signal Processing, vol. 3, pp. 1513–1516 (1998)
8. Cohen, J.: A coefficient of agreement for nominal scales. Educ. Psychol. Measur. **20**(1), 37–46 (1960)
9. Cover, T.M., Thomas, J.A.: Elements of Information Theory. Wiley, New York (2012)
10. Daubechies, I.: Ten Lectures on Wavelets. Society for Industrial and Applied Mathematics, Philadelphia (2006)
11. Dornhege, G.: Toward Brain-Computer Interfacing. The MIT Press, Cambridge (2007)
12. Mallat, S.G.: A theory for multiresolution signal decomposition: the wavelet representation. IEEE Trans. Pattern Anal. Mach. Intell. **11**(7), 674–693 (1989)
13. Martinez-Enriquez, E., Ortega, A.: Lifting transforms on graphs for video coding. In: Data Compression Conference, pp. 73–82. IEEE (2011)
14. Narang, S.K., Ortega, A.: Lifting based wavelet transforms on graphs. In: Conference of Asia-Pacific Signal and Information Processing Association, pp. 441–444 (2009)
15. Peng, H., Long, F., Ding, C.: Feature selection based on mutual information criteria of max-dependency, max-relevance, and min-redundancy. IEEE Trans. Pattern Anal. Mach. Intell. **27**(8), 1226–1238 (2005)
16. Perseh, B., Sharafat, A.R.: An efficient P300-based bci using wavelet features and IBPSO-based channel selection. J. Med. Signals Sens. **2**(3), 128 (2012)
17. Pfurtscheller, G., Lopes da Silva, F.H.: Event-related EEG/MEG synchronization and desynchronization: basic principles. Clin. Neurophysiol. **110**(11), 1842–1857 (1999)
18. Qin, L., He, B.: A wavelet-based timefrequency analysis approach for classification of motor imagery for braincomputer interface applications. J. Neural Eng. **2**, 65 (2005)
19. Ramoser, H., Muller-Gerking, J., Pfurtscheller, G.: Optimal spatial filtering of single trial EEG during imagined hand movement. IEEE Trans. Rehabil. Eng. **8**(4), 441–446 (2000)
20. Schrder, P., Sweldens, W.: Spherical wavelets: Efficiently representing functions on the sphere. In: Proceedings of the 22nd Annual Conference on Computer Graphics and Interactive Techniques, pp. 161–172. ACM (1995)
21. Shen, G., Ortega, A.: Comopact image representation using wavelet lifting along arbitrary trees. In: 15th IEEE International Conference on Image Processing, ICIP 2008, pp. 2808–2811. IEEE (2008)

22. Sweldens, W.: Wavelets and the lifting scheme: a 5 minute tour. Zeitschrift fur Angewandte Mathematik und Mechanik **76**(2), 41–44 (1996)
23. Sweldens, W.: The lifting scheme: a construction of second generation wavelets. SIAM J. Math. Anal. **29**(2), 511 (1998)
24. Sweldens, W., Schrder, P.: Building your own wavelets at home. In: Klees, R., Haagmans, R. (eds.) Wavelets in the Geosciences, pp. 72–107. Springer, Heidelberg (2000)
25. Wu, Z., Yao, D.: Frequency detection with stability coefficient for steady-state visual evoked potential (SSVEP)-based BCIs. J. Neural Eng. **5**(1), 36 (2008)
26. Yong, Y.P.A., Hurley, N.J., Silvestre, G.C.M.: Single-trial EEG classification for brain-computer interface using wavelet decomposition. In: European Signal Processing Conference (EUSIPCO) (2005)

Extracting Emotions
and Communication Styles from Prosody

Licia Sbattella, Luca Colombo$^{(\boxtimes)}$, Carlo Rinaldi, Roberto Tedesco,
Matteo Matteucci, and Alessandro Trivilini

Dip. di Elettronica, Informazione e Biongegneria,
Politecnico di Milano, P.zza Leonardo da Vinci 32, Milano, Italy
{licia.sbattella,roberto.tedesco,matteo.matteucci,
alessandro.trivilini}@polimi.it,
luca.colombo@chem.polimi.it

Abstract. According to many psychological and social studies, vocal messages contain two distinct channels—an explicit, linguistic channel, and an implicit, paralinguistic channel. In particular, the latter contains information about the emotional state of the speaker, providing clues about the implicit meaning of the message. Such information can improve applications requiring human-machine interactions (for example, Automatic Speech Recognition systems or Conversational Agents), as well as support the analysis of human-human interactions (for example, clinic or forensic applications). PrEmA, the tool we present in this work, is able to recognize and classify both emotions and communication style of the speaker, relying on prosodic features. In particular, recognition of communication-styles is, to our knowledge, new, and could be used to infer interesting clues about the state of the interaction. PrEmA uses two LDA-based classifiers, which rely on two sets of prosodic features. Experimenting PrEmA with Italian speakers we obtained $Ac = 71\,\%$ for emotions and $Ac = 86\,\%$ for communication styles.

Keywords: Natural language processing · Communication style recognition · Emotion recognition

1 Introduction

Many psychological and sociological studies highlighted the two distinct channels we use to exchange information among us—a *linguistic* (i.e., explicit) channel used to transmit the contents of a conversation, and a *paralinguistic* (i.e., implicit) channel responsible for providing clues about the emotional state of the speaker and the implicit meaning of the message.

Information conveyed by the paralinguistic channel, in particular prosody, is useful for many research fields where the study of the rhythmic and intonational properties of speech is required [29]. The ability to guess the emotional state of the speaker, as well as her/his communication style, are particularly interesting for Conversational Agents, as could allow them to select the more appropriate

© Springer-Verlag Berlin Heidelberg 2014
H.P. da Silva et al. (Eds.): PhyCS 2014, LNCS 8908, pp. 21–42, 2014.
DOI: 10.1007/978-3-662-45686-6_2

reaction to the user's requests, making the conversation more natural and thus improving the effectiveness of the system [35, 39]. Moreover, being able to extract paralinguistic information is interesting in clinic application, where psychological profiles of subjects and the clinical relationships they establish with doctors could be created. Finally, in forensic applications, paralinguistic information could be useful for observing how defendants, witnesses, and victims behave under interrogation.

Our contribution lies in the latter research field; in particular, we explore techniques for emotion and communication style recognition. In this paper we present an original model, a prototype (PrEmA - Prosodic Emotion Analyzer), and the results we obtained.

The paper is structured as follow. In Sect. 2 we provide a brief introduction about the relationship among voice, emotions, and communication styles; in Sect. 3 we present some research projects about emotion recognition; in Sect. 4 we introduce our model; in Sect. 5 we illustrate the experiments we conducted, and discuss the results we gathered; in Sect. 6 we introduce PrEmA, the prototype we built; finally, in Sect. 7 we draw some conclusions and outline our future research directions.

2   Background

2.1   The Prosodic Elements

Several studies investigate the issue of characterizing human behaviors through vocal expressions; such studies rely on prosodic elements that transmit essential information about the speaker's attitude, emotion, intention, context, gender, age, and physical condition [3, 12, 49].

Intonation makes spoken language very different from written language. In written language, white spaces and punctuation are used to separate words, sentences and phrases, inducing a particular "rhythm" to the sentences. Punctuation also contributes to specify the meaning to the whole sentence, stressing words, creating emphasis on certain parts of the sentence, etc. In spoken language, a similar task is done by means of *prosody*—changes in speech rate, duration of syllables, intonation, loudness, etc.

Such so-called *suprasegmental* characteristics play an important role in the process of utterance understanding; they are key elements in expressing the *intention* of a message (interrogative, affirmative, etc.) and its *style* (aggressive, assertive, etc.) In this work we focused on the following prosodic characteristics [37]: intonation, loudness, duration, pauses, timbre, and rhythm.

intonation (or *tonal variation*, or *melodic contour*) is the most important prosodic effects, and determines the evolution of speech melody. Intonation is tightly related to the illocutionary force of the utterance (e.g., assertion, direction, commission, expression, or declaration). For example, in Italian intonation is the sole way to distinguish among requests (by raising the intonation of the final part of the sentence), assertions (ascending intonation at the beginning of the sentence, then descending intonation in the final part), and commands (descending intonation); thus, it is possible to distinguish the question "vieni domani?" (are you coming tomorrow?) from the assertion "vieni domani" (you are coming tomorrow) or the imperative "vieni domani!" (come tomorrow!).

Moreover, intonation provides clues on the distribution of information in the utterance. In other words, it helps in emphasizing new or important facts the speaker is introducing in the discourse (for example, in Italian, by means of a peak in the intonation contour). Thus, intonation takes part in clarifying the syntactic structure of the utterance.

Finally, and most important for our work, intonation is also related to emotions; for example, the melodic contour of anger is rough and full of sudden variations on accented syllables, while joy exhibits a smooth, rounded, and slow-varying intonation. Intonation also conveys the attitude of the speaker, leading the hearer to grasp nuances of meaning, like irony, kindness, impatience, etc.

loudness is another important prosodic feature, and is directly related to the voice loudness. Loudness can emphasize differences in terms of meaning—an increase of loudness, for example, can be related to anger.

duration (or *speech rate*) indicates the length of phonetic segments. Duration can transmit a wide range of meanings, such as speaker's emotions; in general, emotional states that imply psychophysiological activation (like fear, anger, and joy) are correlated to short durations and high speech rate [10], while sadness is typically related to slow speech. Duration also correlates with the speaker's attitudes (it gives clues about courtesy, impatience, or insecurity of the speaker), as well as types of discourse (a homily will have slower speech rate than, for example, a sport running commentary).

pauses allow the speaker to take breath, but can also be used to emphasize parts of the utterance, by inserting breaks in the intonation contour; from this point of view, pauses correspond to punctuation we add in written language. Pauses, however, are much more general and can convey a larger variety of nuances than punctuation.

timbre –such as falsetto, whisper, hoarse voice, quavering voice– often provide information about the emotional state and health of the speaker (for example, a speaker feeling insecure is easily associated with quavering voice). Timbre also depends on the mount of noise affecting the vocal emission.

rhythm is a complex prosodic element, emerging from joint action of several factors, in particular intonation, loudness, and duration. It is an intrinsic and unique attribute of each language.

In the following, we present some studies that try to model the relationship among prosody, emotions, and communication styles.

2.2 Speech and Emotions

Emotion is a complex construct and represents a component of how we react to external stimuli [44]. In emotions we can distinguish:

- A neurophysiological component of activation (arousal).
- A cognitive component, through which an individual evaluates the situation-stimulus in relation to her/his needs.
- A motoric component, which aims at transforming intentions in actions.
- An expressive component, through which an individual expresses her/his intentions in relation to her/his level of social interaction.
- A subjective component, which is related to the experience of the individual.

The emotional expression is not only based on linguistic events, but also on paralinguistic events, which can be acoustic (such as screams or particular vocal inflections), visual (such as facial expressions or gestures), tactile (for example, a caress), gustatory, olfactory, and motoric [5,38]. In particular, the contribution of non-verbal channels on the communication process is huge; according to [33] the linguistic, paralinguistic, and motoric channels, constitutes, respectively, 7%, 38%, and 55% of the communication process. In this work, we focused on the acoustic paralinguistic channel.

According to [48], emotions can be divided in: *vital affects* (floating, vanishing, spending, exploding, increasing, decreasing, bloated, exhausted, etc.) and *categorical affects* (happiness, sadness, anger, fear, disgust, surprise, interest, shame). The former are very difficult to define and recognize, while the latter can be more easily treated. Thus, in this work we focused on categorical affects.

Finally, emotions have two components—an *hedonic tone*, which refers to the degree of pleasure, or displeasure, connected to the emotion; and an *activation*, which refers to the intensity of the physiological activation [30]. In this work we relied on the latter component, which is easier to measure.

Classifying Emotions. Several well-known theories for classifying emotions have been proposed. In [41] authors consider a huge number of characteristics about emotions, identifying two primary axes: pleasantness/unpleasantness and arousal/inhibition.

In [24] the author lists 10 primary emotions: sadness, joy, surprise, sadness, anger, disgust, contempt, fear, shame, guilt; in [50] the latest one is eliminated; in [17] a more restrictive classification (happiness, surprise, fear, sadness, anger, disgust) is proposed.

In particular, Ekman distinguishes between *primary emotions*, quickly activated and difficult to control (for example, anger, fear, disgust, happiness, sadness, surprise), and *secondary emotions*, which undergo social control and cognitive filtering (for example, shame, jealousy, pride). In this work we focused on primary emotions.

Mapping Speech and Emotions. As stated before, voice is considered a very reliable indicator of emotional states. The relationship between voice and emotion is based on the assumption that the physiological responses typical of an emotional state, such as the modification of breathing, phonation and articulation of sounds, produce detectable changes in the acoustic indexes associated to the production of speech.

Several theories have been developed in an effort to find a correlation among speech characteristics and emotions. For example, for Italian [2]:

- Fear is expressed as a subtle, tense, and tight tone.
- Sadness is communicated using a low tone, with the presence of long pauses and slow speech rate.
- Joy is expressed with a very sharp tone and with a progressive intonation profile, with increasing loudness and, sometimes, with an acceleration in speech rate.

In [1] it is suggested that active emotions produce faster speech, with higher frequencies and wider loudness range, while the low-activation emotions are associated with slow voice and low frequencies.

In [25] the author proposes a detailed study of the relationship between emotion an prosodic characteristics. His approach is based on time, loudness, spectrum, attack, articulation, and differences in duration [26]. Table 1 shows such prosodic characterization, for the four primary emotions; our work started from such clues, trying to derive measurable acoustic features.

Relying on the aforementioned works, we decided to focus on the following emotions: *joy*, *fear*, *anger*, *sadness*, and *neutral*.

2.3   Speech and Communication Styles

The process of communication has been studied from many points of view. Communication not only conveys information and expresses emotions, it is also characterized by a particular relational style (i.e., a *communication style*). Everyone has a relational style that, from time to time, may be more or less dominant or passive, sociable or withdrawn, aggressive or friendly, welcoming or rejecting.

Classifying Communication Styles. We chose to rely on the following simple classification and description that includes three communication styles [34]: *passive*, *assertive*, and *aggressive*.

Passive communication imply not expressing honest feelings, thoughts and beliefs. Therefore, allowing others to violate your rights; expressing thoughts and feelings in an apologetic, self-effacing way, so that others easily disregard them; sometimes showing a subtle lack of respect for the other person's ability to take disappointments, shoulder some responsibility, or handle their own problems.

Persons with aggressive communication style stand up for their personal rights and express their thoughts, feelings and beliefs in a way which is usually inappropriate and always violates the rights of the other person. They tend to maintain their superiority by putting others down. When threatened, they tend to attack.

Finally, assertive communication is a way of communicating feelings, thoughts, and beliefs in an open, honest manner without violating the rights of others. It is an alternative to being aggressive where we abuse other people's rights, and passive where we abuse our own rights.

Table 1. Prosodic characterization of emotions

Emotion	Prosodic feature
Joy	- quick meters
	- moderate duration variations
	- high average sound level
	- tendency to tighten up the contrasts between long and short words
	- articulation predominantly detached
	- quick attacks
	- brilliant tone
	- slight or missing vibrato
	- slightly rising intonation
Sadness	- slow meter
	- relatively large variations in duration
	- low noise level
	- tendency to attenuate the contrasts between long and short words
	- articulation linked
	- soft attacks
	- slow and wide vibrato
	- final delaying
	- soft tone
	- intonation (at times) slightly declining
Anger	- quick meters
	- high noise level
	- relatively sharp contrasts between long and short words
	- articulation mostly not linked
	- very dry attacks
	- sharply stamp
	- distorted notes
Fear	- quick meters
	- high noise level
	- relatively sharp contrasts between long and short words
	- articulation mostly not linked
	- very dry attacks
	- sharply stamp
	- distorted notes

Mapping Speech and Communication Styles. Starting from the aforementioned characteristics of communication styles, considering the prosodic clues provided in [34], and taking into account other works [20–22,46,47], we came out with the prosodic characterization showed in Table 2.

Table 2. Prosodic characterization of communication styles

Communication style	Prosodic feature
Passive	- flickering
	- voice often dull and monoto-nous
	- tone may be sing-song or whining
	- low Volume
	- hesitant, filled with pauses
	- slow-fast or fast-slow
	- frequent throat clearing
Aggressive	- very firm voice
	- often abrupt, clipped
	- often fast
	- tone sarcastic, cold, harsh
	- grinding
	- fluent, without hesitations
	- voice can be strident, often shouting, rising at end
Assertive	- firm, relaxed voice
	- steady even pace
	- tone is middle range, rich and warm
	- not over-loud or quiet
	- fluent, few hesitation

2.4   Acoustic Features

As we discussed above, characterizing emotional states and communication styles associated to a vocal signal implies measuring some acoustic features, which, in turn, are derived from physiological reactions. Tables 1 and 2 provide some clues about how to relate such physiological reactions to prosodic characteristics, but we need to define a set of measurable acoustic features.

Acoustic Features for Emotions. We started from the most studied acoustic features [14,31,36,51]:

pitch measures the intonation, and is represented by the fundamental harmonic (F0); it tends to increase for anger, joy, and fear; it decreases for sadness. Pitch tends to be more variable for anger and joy.

intensity represents the amplitude of the vocal signal, and measures the loudness; intensity tends to increase for anger and joy, decrease for sadness, and stay constant for fear.

time measures duration and pauses, as voiced and unvoiced segments. High speech rate is associated to anger, joy, and fear while low speech rate is associated to sadness. Irregular speech rate is often associated with anger and sadness. Time is also an important parameter for distinguishing articulation breaks (speaker's breathing) from *unvoiced* segments. The unvoiced segments represent *silences*—parts of the signal where the information of the pitch and/or intensity are below a certain threshold.

voice quality measures the timbre and is related to variations of the voice spectrum, as to the signal-noise ratio. In particular:

- Changes in amplitude of the waveform between successive cycles (called *shimmer*).
- Changes in the frequency of the waveform between successive cycles (called *jitter*).
- Hammarberg's index, which covers the difference between the energy in the 0–2000 Hz and 2000–5000 Hz bands.
- The harmonic/noise ratio (HNR) between the energy of the harmonic part of the signal and the remaining part of the signal; see [6,18,19].

High values of shimmer and jitter characterize, for example, disgust and sadness, while fear and joy are distinguished by different values of the Hammarberg's index.

Acoustic Features for Communication Styles. Starting from clues provided by Table 2, we decided to rely on the same acoustic features we used for the emotion recognition (pitch, intensity, time, and voice quality). But, in order to recognize complex prosodic variations that particularly affects communication style, we reviewed the literature and found that research mostly focuses on the variations of tonal accents within a sentence and at a level of prominent syllables [4,15,16]. Thus, we added two more elements to our acoustic feature set:

- Contour of the pitch curve.
- Contour of the intensity curve.

In Sect. 4.2 we will show how we measured the feature set we defined for emotions and communication style.

3   Related Work

Several approaches exist in literature for the task of emotion recognition, based on classifiers like Support Vector Machines (SVM), decision trees, Neural Networks (NN), etc. In the following, we present some of such approaches.

The system described in [27] made use of SVM for classifying emotions expressed by a group of professional speakers. The authors underlined that, for extreme emotions (anger, happiness and fear), the most useful information was contained in the first words of the sentence, while last words were more discriminative in case of neutral emotion. The recognition Precision[1] of the system, on average, using prosodic parameters and considering only the beginning words, was around 36 %.

The approach described in [11] used SVM, too, applying it to the German language. In particular, this project developed a prototype for analyzing the mood of customers in call centers. This research showed that pitch and intensity were the most important features for the emotional speech, while features on spectral energy distribution were the most important voice quality features. Recognition Precision they obtained was, on average, around 70 %.

Another approach leveraged the Alternating Decision Trees (ADTree), for the analysis of humorous spoken conversations from a classic comedy TV show [40]; speaker turns were classified as humorous or non-humorous. They used a combination of prosodic (e.g., pitch, energy, duration, silences, etc.) and non-prosodic features (e.g., words, turn length, etc.) Authors discovered that the best set of features was related to the gender of the speaker. Their classifier obtained Accuracies of 64.63 % for males and 64.8 % for females.

The project described in [45] made use of NN. The project used two databases of Chinese utterances. One was composed of speech recorded by non-professional speakers, while the other was composed of TV recordings. They used Mel-Frequency Cepstral Coefficients, considering six speech emotions: angry, happiness, sadness, and surprised. They obtained the following Precisions: angry 66 %, happiness 57.8 %, sadness 85.1 %, and surprised 58.7 %.

The approaches described in [28] used a combination of three different sources of information: acoustic, lexical, and discourse. They proposed a case study for detecting negative and non-negative emotions using spoken language coming from a call center application. In particular, the samples were obtained from real users involved in spoken dialog with an automatic agent over the telephone. In order to capture the emotional features at the lexical level, they introduced a new concept named "emotional salience"—an emotionally salient word, with respect to a category, tends to appear more often in that category than in other categories. For the acoustic analysis they compared a K-Nearest Neighborhood classifier and a Linear Discriminant Classifier. The results of the project demonstrated that the best performance was obtained when acoustic and language features were combined. The best performing results of this project, in terms of classification errors, were 10.65 % for males and 7.95 % for females.

Finally, in [23] authors focuses on "emotional temperature" (ET) as a biomarker for early Alzheimer disease detection. They leverages non linear features, such as the Fractal Dimension, and rely on a SVM for classifying ET of voice frames as pathological or non-pathological. They claim an Accuracy of 90.7 % to 97.7 %.

---

[1] Notice that the performance index provided in this section are indicative and cannot be compared each other, since each system used its own vocal dataset.

Our project is based on classifiers that leverage the Linear Discriminant Analysis (LDA) [32]; such a model is simpler than SVM and NN, and easier to train. Moreover, with respect to approaches making use of textual features, our model is considerably simpler. Nevertheless, our approach provides good results (see Sect. 5).

Finally, we didn't find any system able to classify communication styles so, to our knowledge, this feature provided by our system is novel.

4   The Model

For each voiced segment, two set of features –one for recognizing emotions and one for communication style– were calculated; then, by means of two LDA-based classifiers, such segments were associated with emotion and communication style.

LDA-based classifier provided a good trade-off between performance and classification correctness. LDA projects vectors of features, which represents the samples to analyze, to a smaller space. The method maximizes the ratio of between-class variance to the within-class variance, permitting to maximize class separability. More formally, LDA finds the eigenvectors ϕ_i that solve:

$$\mathbf{B}\phi_i - \lambda\mathbf{W}\phi_i = 0 \tag{1}$$

where $\mathbf{B}$ is the between-class scatter matrix and $\mathbf{W}$ is the within-class scatter matrix. Once a sample $\boldsymbol{x}_j$ is projected on the new space provided by the eigenvectors, the class $\hat{k}$ corresponding to the projection $\boldsymbol{y}_j$ is chosen according to [9]:

$$\hat{k} = \operatorname*{argmax}_k p(k|\boldsymbol{y}_j) = \operatorname*{argmax}_k -d_k^2(\boldsymbol{y}_j) \tag{2}$$

where $d_k^2(\cdot)$ is the generalized squared distance function:

$$d_k^2(\boldsymbol{y}) = (\boldsymbol{y} - \boldsymbol{\mu}_j)^T \Sigma_k^{-1}(\boldsymbol{y} - \boldsymbol{\mu}_j) + \frac{\ln|\Sigma_k|}{2} - \ln p(k) \tag{3}$$

where Σ_k is the covariance matrix for the class k and $p(k)$ is the a-priori probability of the class k:

$$p(k) = \frac{n_k}{\sum_{i=1}^{K} n_i} \tag{4}$$

where n_k is the number of samples belonging to the class k, and K is the number of classes.

4.1   Creating a Corpus

Our model was trained and tested on a corpus of sentences, labeled with the five basic emotions and the three communication styles we introduced. We collected 900 sentences, uttered by six Italian professional speakers, asking them to simulate emotions and communication styles. This way, we obtained good samples, showing clear emotions and expressing the desired communication styles.

4.2 Measuring and Selecting Acoustic Features

Figure 1 shows the activities that lead to the calculation of the acoustic features: Preprocessing, segmentation, and feature extraction. The result is the dataset we used for training and testing the classifiers.

In the following, the aforementioned phases are presented. The values shown for the various parameters needed by the voice-processing routines, have been chosen experimentally (see Sect. 4.3 for details on how the values of such parameters were selected; see Sect. 6 for details on Praat, the voice-processing tool we adopted).

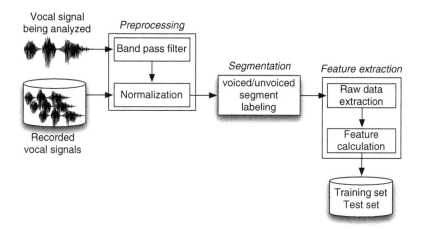

Fig. 1. The feature calculation process

Preprocessing and Segmentation. We used a Hann band filter, for removing useless harmonics ($F_{Lo} = 100\,$Hz, $F_{Hi} = 6\,$kHz, and smoothing $w = 100\,$Hz). Then, we normalized the intensity of different audio files, so that the average intensity of different recordings was uniform and matched a predefined setpoint. Finally, we divided the audio signal into *segments*; in particular we divided *voiced segments*, where the average, normalized intensity was above the threshold $I_{voicing} = 0.45$, and *silenced segments*, where the average, normalized intensity was below the threshold $I_{silence} = 0.03$. Segments having average, normalized intensity between the two thresholds were not considered[2].

Feature Calculation. For features related to Pitch, we used the following range $F_{floor} = 75\,$Hz, $F_{ceiling} = 600\,$Hz (such values are well suited for male voices, as we used male subjects for our experiments).

---

[2] Such segments were considered too loud for being clear silences, but too quiet for providing a clear voiced signal.

Among features related with Time, *articulation ratio* refers to the amount of time taken by voiced segments, excluding articulation breaks, divided by the total recording time; an *articulation break* is a pause –in a voiced segment– longer than a given threshold (we used the threshold $T_{break} = 0.25\,s$), and is used to capture the speaker's breathing. The *speech ratio*, instead, is the percentage of voiced segments over the total recording time. These two parameters are very similar for short utterances, because articulation breaks are negligible; for long utterances, however, these parameters definitely differ, revealing that articulation breaks are an intrinsic property of the speaker. Finally, *unvoiced frame ratio* is the total time of unvoiced frames, divided by the recording total time.

The speech signal, even if produced with maximum stationarity, contains variations of F0 and intensity [19]; such variations represents the perceived voice quality. The random changes in the short term (micro disturbances) of F0 are defined as *jitter*, while the variations of the amplitude are known as *shimmer*. The Harmonic-to-Noise ratio (HNR) value is the "degree of hoarseness" of the signal—the extent to which noise replaces the harmonic structure in the spectrogram [7].

Finally, the following features represent Pitch and Intensity contours:

– Pitch contour
  - Number of peaks per second. The number of maxima in the pitch contour, within a voiced segment, divided by the duration of the segment.
  - Average and variance of peak values.
  - Average gradient. The average gradient between two consecutive sampling points in the pitch curve.
  - Variance of gradients. The variance of such pitch gradients.
– Intensity contour
  - Number of peaks per second. The number of maxima in the intensity curve, within a voiced segment, divided by the duration of the segment.
  - Mean and variance of peak values.
  - Variance of peak values.
  - Average gradient. The average gradient between two consecutive sampling points in the intensity curve.
  - Variance of gradients. The variance of such intensity gradients.

Tables 3 and 4 summarized the acoustic features we measured, for emotions and communication styles, respectively.

Feature Selection. In order to obtain the minimum feature set, we used the ANOVA and LSD tests to discard highly correlated measurements.

The ANOVA analysis for features related to emotions (assuming 0.01 as significance threshold) found all the features to be significant, except Average_Intensity. For Average_intensity we leveraged the Fischer's LSD test, which showed that Average_Intensity was not useful for discriminating Joy from Neutral and Sadness, Neutral from Sadness, and Fear from Anger. Nevertheless Average_Intensity was retained, as LSD proved it useful for discriminating Sadness, Joy, and Neutral from Anger and Fear.

Table 3. Measured acoustic features for emotions

Features	Characteristics
Pitch (F0)	Average [Hz]
	Standard deviation [Hz]
	Maximum [Hz]
	Minimum [Hz]
	25th quantile [Hz]
	75th quantile [Hz]
	Median [Hz]
Intensity	Average [dB]
	Standard deviation [dB]
	Maximum [dB]
	Minimum [dB]
	Median [dB]
Time	Unvoiced frame ratio [%]
	Articulation break ratio [%]
	Articulation ratio [%]
	Speech ratio [%]
Voice quality	Jitter [%]
	Shimmer [%]
	HNR [dB]

The ANOVA analysis for features related to communication style (assuming 0.01 as significance threshold) found eight potentially useless features: Average_Intensity, 90_th_quantile, Unvoiced_frame_ratio, Peaks_per_second, Average_peak_gradient, Standard_deviation_peaks_gradient, Median_intensity, and Standard_deviation_intensity. For such features we performed the LSD test, which showed that Peaks_per_second was not able to discriminate Aggressive vs Assertive, but was useful for discriminating all others communication styles and thus we decided to retain it. The others seven features were dropped as LSD showed that they were not useful for discriminating communication styles.

After this selection, the set of features for the emotion recognition task remained unchanged, while the set of features for the communication-style recognition task was reduced (in Table 4, text in italics indicates removed features).

4.3   Training

The Vocal Dataset. For the creation of the vocal corpus we examined the public vocal databases available for the Italian language (EUROM0, EUROM1 and AIDA), public audiobooks, and different resources provided by professional actors. After a detailed evaluation of available resources, we realized that they

Table 4. Measured acoustic features for communication style (features in italics were removed by means of the ANOVA/LSD analysis)

Features	Characteristics
Pitch (F0)	Average [Hz]
	Standard deviation [Hz]
	Maximum [Hz]
	Minimum [Hz]
	10th quantile [Hz]
	90th quantile [Hz]
	Median [Hz]
Pitch contour	Peaks per second [#peaks/s]
	Average peaks height [Hz]
	Variance of peak heights [Hz]
	Average peak gradient [Hz/s]
	Variance of peak gradients [Hz/s]
Intensity	*Average [dB]*
	Standard deviation [dB]
	Maximum [dB]
	Minimum [dB]
	10th quantile [dB]
	90th quantile [dB]
	Median [dB]
Intensity contour	Peaks per second [#peaks/s]
	Average peak height [dB]
	Variance of peaks heights [dB]
	Average peak gradients [dB/s]
	Variance of peak gradients [dB/s]
Time	*Unvoiced frame ratio [%]*
	Articulation break ratio [%]
	Articulation ratio [%]
	Speech ratio [%]
Voice quality	Jitter [%]
	Shimmer [%]
	NHR [dB]

were not suitable for our study, due to the scarcity of sequences where emotion an communication style were unambiguously expressed.

We therefore opted for the development of our own datasets, composed of:

– A series of sentences, with different emotional intentions.
– A series of monologues, with different communication styles.

We carefully selected –taking into account the work presented in [13]– 10 sentences for each emotion, expressing strong and clear emotional states. This way, it was easier for the actor to communicate the desired emotional state, because the meaning of the sentence already contained the emotional intention. With the same approach we selected 3 monologues (about ten to fifteen rows long, each)—they were chosen to help the actor in identifying himself with the desired communication style.

For example, to represent the passive style we chose some monologues by Woody Allen; to represent the aggressive style, we chose "The night before the trial" by Anton Chekhov; and to represent assertive style, we used the book "Redesigning the company" by Richard Normann.

We selected six male actors; each one was recorded independently and individually, in order to avoid mutual conditioning. In addition, each actor received the texts in advance, in order to review them and practice before the registration.

The Learning Process. The first step of the learning process was to select the parameters needed by the voice-processing routines. Using the whole vocal dataset we trained several classifiers, varying the parameters, and selected the best combination according to the performance indexes we defined (see Sect. 5). We did it for both the emotion recognition classifier and the communication style recognition classifier, obtaining two parameter sets.

Once the parameter sets were defined, a subset of the vocal dataset –the training dataset– was used to train the two classifiers. In particular, for the emotional dataset –containing 900 voiced segments– and the communication-style dataset –containing 54 paragraphs– we defined a training dataset containing 90 % of the initial dataset, and an evaluation dataset with the remaining 10 %.

Then, we trained the two classifiers on the training dataset. Such process was repeated 10 times, with different training set/test set subdivisions.

5   Evaluation and Discussion

During the evaluation phase, the 10 pairs of LDA-based classifiers we trained (10 for emotions and 10 for communication styles) tagged each voiced segment in the evaluation dataset with an emotion and an communication style. Then performance metrics were calculated for each classifier; finally, average performance metrics were calculated (see Sect. 6 for details on Praat, the voice-processing tool we adopted).

5.1 Emotions

The validation dataset consists of 18 voiced segments chosen at random for each of the five emotions, for a total of 90 voiced segments (10 % of the whole emotion dataset).

The average performance indexes of the 10 trained classifiers, are shown in Tables 5 and 6.

Table 5. Confusion matrix for emotions (%)

	Predicted emotions				
	Joy	Neutral	Fear	Anger	Sadness
Joy	**63.81**	0.00	18.35	11.79	6.05
Neutral	3.47	**77.51**	2.14	1.79	15.09
Fear	33.75	0.00	**58.35**	6.65	1.25
Anger	10.24	1.16	8.16	**77.28**	3.16
Sadness	5.14	14.44	0.28	0.81	**79.33**

Table 6. Precision, Recall, and F-measure for emotions (%)

	Joy	Neutral	Fear	Anger	Sadness
Pr	56.03	75.00	64.84	80.36	80.28
Re	63.53	76.36	58.42	77.10	79.39
F_1	59.54	75.68	61.46	78.70	79.83

Table 7. Average Pr, Re, F_1, and Ac, for emotions (%)

Avg Pr	71.44
Avg Re	71.06
Avg F_1	71.16
Ac	71.27

Table 8. Error rates for emotions

	Joy	Neutral	Fear	Anger	Sadness
F_p	164	56	96	65	70
F_n	120	52	126	79	74
T_e (%)	**18.25**	**6.94**	**14.27**	**9.25**	**9.25**

Precision and F-measure are good for Neutral, Anger, and Sadness, while Fear and Joy are more problematic (especially Joy, which has the worst value).

The issue is confirmed by the confusion matrix of Table 5, which shows that Joy phrases were tagged as Fear 33 % of the time, lowering the Precision of both. Recall is good for all the emotions and also for Joy, which exhibits the better value. The average values for Precision, Recall, and F-measure are about 71 %; Accuracy exhibits a similar value (see Table 7).

The K value, the agreement between the classifier and the dataset, is $K = 0.64$, meaning a good agreement was found.

Finally, for each class, we calculated false positives F_p (number of voiced segments belonging to another class, incorrectly tagged in the class), false negatives F_n (number of voiced segments belonging to this class, incorrectly classified in another class), and thus the error rate T_e (see Table 8). Joy and Fear exhibit the highest errors, as the classifier often confused them. We argue this result is due to the highs degree of arousal that characterize both Joy and Fear.

5.2   Communication Styles

The validation data set consists of 2 randomly chosen paragraphs, for each of the three communication styles, for a total of 6 paragraphs, which corresponds to 10 % of the communication-style dataset.

The average performance indexes of the 10 trained models, are shown in Tables 9 and 10.

Table 9. Confusion matrix for communication styles (%)

	Predicted communication styles		
	Aggressive	Assertive	Passive
Aggressive	**99.30**	0.70	0.00
Assertive	24.26	**62.68**	13.06
Passive	7.08	10.30	**82.62**

Table 10. Precision, Recall, and F-measure for communication styles (%)

	Aggressive	Assertive	Passive
Pr	85.55	68.32	93.61
Re	99.33	60.53	83.25
F_1	91.93	64.19	88.13

Precision, Recall, and F-measure indicate very good performances for Aggressive and Passive communication styles; acceptable but much smaller values are obtained for Assertive sentences, as they are often tagged as Aggressive (24.26 % of the time, as shown in the confusion matrix). The average values for Precision, Recall, and F-measure are about 86 %; Accuracy exhibits a similar value (see Table 11).

Table 11. Average Pr, Re, F_1, and Ac, for communication-style (%)

Avg Pr	86.10
Avg Re	85.87
Avg F_1	85.61
Ac	86.00

Table 12. Error rate for communication style

	Aggressive	Assertive	Passive
F_p	100	64	36
F_n	4	90	106
T_e (%)	**7.14**	**10.57**	**9.75**

The K value, the agreement between the classifier and the dataset, is $K = 0.78$, meaning that a good agreement was found.

Finally, Table 12 shows error rates for each class. As expected, Assertive exhibits the highest error (10.57 %), while the best result is achieved by the recognition of Aggressive, with an error rate of 7.14 %. Analyzing the F_p and F_n values we noted that only Aggressive had $F_n > F_p$, which means that the classifier tended to mistakenly associate such a class to segments where it was not appropriate.

6　The Prototype

The application architecture is composed of five modules (see Fig. 2): GUI, Feature Extraction, Emotion Recognition, Communication-style Recognition, and Praat.

Praat [8] is a well-known open-source tool for speech analysis[3]; it provides several functionalities for the analysis of vocal signals as well as a statistical module (containing the LDA-based classifier we described in Sect. 4). The scripting functionalities provided by Praat permitted us to quickly implement our prototype.

The GUI module permits to choose the audio file to analyze, and shows the results to the user; the Feature Extraction module performs the calculations presented in Sect. 4 (preprocessing, segmentation, and feature calculation); the Emotion Recognition and Communication-style Recognition modules rely on the two best-performing[4] models to classify the input file according to its emotional

---

[3] http://www.fon.hum.uva.nl/praat/.

[4] From the 10 LDA-based classifiers generated for the emotion classification task, the one with better performance indexes was chosen as a final model; the same approach was followed for the communication-style classifier.

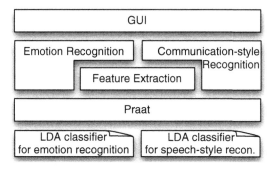

Fig. 2. The PrEmA architecture overview

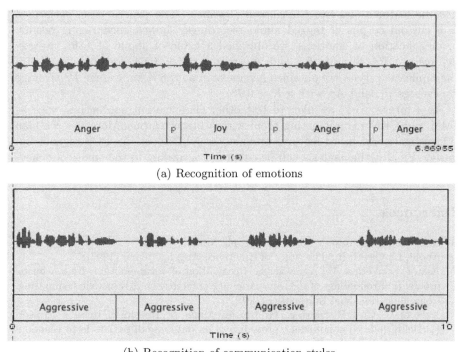

(a) Recognition of emotions

(b) Recognition of communication styles

Fig. 3. Recognition of emotions and communication styles

state and communication style. All the calculations are implemented by means of scripts that leverage functionalities provided by Praat.

Figure 3 shows two screenshots of the PrEmA application (translated in English) recognizing, respectively, emotions and communication styles. In particular, in Fig. 3(a) the application analyzed a sentence of 6.87 s expressing anger, divided in four segments (i.e., three silences where found); each segment was assigned with an emotion: Anger, Joy (mistakenly), Anger, Anger. Figure 3(b) shows the first 10 s fragment of a 123.9 s aggressive speech; the application found 40 segments and assigned them with a communication style (in the example, the segments where all classified as Aggressive).

7   Conclusion and Future Work

We presented PrEmA, a tool able to recognize emotions and communication styles from vocal signals, providing clues about the state of the conversation. In particular, we consider communication-style recognition as our main contribution since it could provide a potentially powerful mean for understanding user's needs, problems and desires.

The tool, written using the Praat scripting language, relies on two sets of prosodic features and two LDA-based classifiers. The experiments, performed on a custom corpus of tagged audio recordings, showed encouraging results: for classification of emotions, we obtained a value of about 71 % for average Pr, average Re, average F_1, and Ac, with a $K = 0.64$; for classification of communication styles, we obtained a value of about 86 % for average Pr, average Re, average F_1, and Ac, with a $K = 0.78$.

As a future work, we plan to test other classification approaches, such as HMM and CRF, experimenting them with a bigger corpus. Moreover, we plan to investigate text-based features provided by NLP tools, like POS taggers and parsers. Finally, the analysis will be enhanced according to the "musical behavior" methodology [42, 43].

References

1. Anolli, L.: Le emozioni. Edizioni Unicopli, Milano (2002)
2. Anolli, L., Ciceri, R.: The Voice of Emotions. Angeli, Milano (1997)
3. Asawa, K., Verma, V., Agrawal, A.: Recognition of vocal emotions from acoustic profile. In: Proceedings of the International Conference on Advances in Computing, Communications and Informatics (2012)
4. Avesani, C., Cosi, P., Fauri, E., Gretter, R., Mana, N., Rocchi, S., Rossi, F., Tesser, F.: Definizione ed annotazione prosodica di un database di parlato-letto usando il formalismo ToBI. In: Proceedings of Il Parlato Italiano, Napoli, Italy, February 2003
5. Balconi, M., Carrera, A.: Il lessico emotivo nel decoding delle espressioni facciali. ESE - Psychofenia - Salento University Publishing (2005)
6. Banse, R., Sherer, K.R.: Acoustic profiles in vocal emotion expression. J. Pers. Soc. Psychol. **70**, 614–636 (1996)
7. Boersma, P.: Accurate short-term analysis of the fundamental frequency and the Harmonics-to-Noise ratio of a sampled sound. In: Proceedings of Institute of Phonetic Sciences, University of Amsterdam, vol. 17, pp. 97–110 (1993). http://www.fon.hum.uva.nl/paul/papers/Proceedings_1993.pdf
8. Boersma, P.: Praat, a system for doing phonetics by computer. Glot Int. **5**(9/10), 341–345 (2001)
9. Boersma, P., Weenink, D.: Manual of praat: doing phonetics by computer [computer program] (2013)

10. Bonvino, E.: Le strutture del linguaggio: un'introduzione alla fonologia. La Nuova Italia, Milano (2000)

11. Borchert, M., Diisterhoft, A.: Emotions in speech - experiments with prosody and quality features in speech for use in categorical and dimensional emotion recognition environments. In: IEEE Natural Language Processing and Knowledge Engineering (2005)

12. Caldognetto, E.M., Poggi, I.: Il parlato emotivo. aspetti cognitivi, linguistici e fonetici. In: Il parlato italiano. Atti del Convegno Nazionale. Napoli, Italy (2004)

13. Canepari, L.: L'intonazione linguistica e paralinguistica. Liguori Editore (1985)

14. Cowie, R., Douglas-Cowie, E., Tsapatsoulis, N., Votsis, G., Kollias, S., Fellenz, W.: Emotion recognition in human-computer interaction. IEEE Signal Process. Mag. **18**(1), 32–80 (2001)

15. D'Anna, L., Petrillo, M.: APA: un prototipo di sistema automatico per l'analisi prosodica. In: Atti delle 11me giornate di studio del Gruppo di Fonetica Sperimentale (2001)

16. Delmonte, R.: SLIM prosodic automatic tools for self-learning instruction. Speech Commun. **30**, 145–166 (2000)

17. Ekman, D., Ekman, P., Davidson, R.: The Nature of Emotion: Fundamental Questions. Oxford University Press, New York, Oxford (1994)

18. Gobl, C., Chasaide, A.N.: Testing affective correlates of voice quality through analysis and resynthesis. In: ISCA Workshop on Emotion and Speech (2000)

19. Hammarberg, B., Fritzell, B., Gauffin, J., Sundberg, J., Wedin, L.: Perceptual and acoustic correlates of voice qualities. Acta Otolaryngol. **90**(1–6), 441–451 (1980)

20. Hastie, H.W., Poesio, M., Isard, S.: Automatically predicting dialog structure using prosodic features. Speech Commun. **36**(1–2), 63–79 (2001)

21. Hirshberg, J., Avesani, C.: Prosodic disambiguation in English and Italian. In: Botinis, A. (ed.) Intonation. Kluwer, Dordrecht (2000)

22. Hirst, D.: Automatic analysis of prosody for multilingual speech corpora. In: Keller, E., Bailly, G., Terken, J., Huckvale, M. (eds.) Improvements in Speech Synthesis. Wiley, Chichester (2001)

23. López-de-Ipiña, K., Alonso, J.B., Travieso, C.M., Solé-Casals, J., Egiraun, H., Faundez-Zanuy, M., Ezeiza, A., Barroso, N., Ecay-Torres, M., Martinez-Lage, P., de Lizardui, U.M.: On the selection of non-invasive methods based on speech analysis oriented to automatic alzheimer disease diagnosis. Sensors **13**(5), 6730–6745 (2013). http://www.mdpi.com/1424-8220/13/5/6730

24. Izard, C.E.: The Face of Emotion. Appleton Century Crofts, New York (1971)

25. Juslin, P.N.: Emotional communication in music performance: a functionalist perspective and some data. Music Percept. **14**(4), 383–418 (1997)

26. Juslin, P.: A Functionalist Perspective on Emotional Communication in Music Performance, 1st edn. Acta Universitatis Upsaliensis, Uppsala (1998)

27. Koolagudi, S.G., Kumar, N., Rao, K.S.: Speech emotion recognition using segmental level prosodic analysis. In: IEEE, Devices and Communications (ICDeCom) (2011)

28. Lee, C.M., Narayanan, S.: Toward detecting emotions in spoken dialogs. IEEE Trans. Speech Audio Process. **13**(2), 293–303 (2005)

29. Leung, C., Lee, T., Ma, B., Li, H.: Prosodic attribute model for spoken language identification. In: IEEE International Conference on Acoustics, Speech and Signal Processing (ICASSP 2010) (2010)

30. Mandler, G.: Mind and Body: Psychology of Emotion and Stress. Norton, New York (1984)

31. McGilloway, S., Cowie, R., Cowie, E.D., Gielen, S., Westerdijk, M., Stroeve, S.: Approaching automatic recognition of emotion from voice: a rough benchmark. In: ISCA Workshop on Speech and Emotion (2000)
32. McLachlan, G.J.: Discriminant Analysis and Statistical Pattern Recognition. Wiley, New York (2004)
33. Mehrabian, A.: Nonverbal Communication. Aldine-Atherton, Chicago (1972)
34. Michel, F.: Assert Yourself. Centre for Clinical Interventions, Perth (2008)
35. Moridis, C.N., Economides, A.A.: Affective learning: empathetic agents with emotional facial and tone of voice expressions. IEEE Trans. Affect. Comput. 3(3) (2012)
36. Murray, E., Arnott, J.L.: Towards a simulation of emotion in synthetic speech: a review of the literature on human vocal emotion. J. Acoust. Soc. Am. 93(2), 1097–1108 (1993)
37. Pinker, S., Prince, A.: Regular and irregular morphology and the psychological status of rules of grammar. In: Lima, S.D., Corrigan, R.L., Iverson, G.K. (eds.) The Reality of Linguistic Rules. John Benjamins Publishing Company, Amsterdam/Philadelphia (1994)
38. Planet, S., Iriondo, I.: Comparison between decision-level and feature-level fusion of acoustic and linguistic features for spontaneous emotion recognition. In: Information Systems and Technologies (CISTI) (2012)
39. Pleva, M., Ondas, S., Juhar, J., Cizmar, A., Papaj, J., Dobos, L.: Speech and mobile technologies for cognitive communication and information systems. In: 2011 2nd International Conference on Cognitive Infocommunications (CogInfoCom), July 2011, pp. 1–5 (2011)
40. Purandare, A., Litman, D.: Humor: Prosody analysis and automatic recognition for F * R * I * E * N * D * S *. In: Proceedings of the Conference on Empirical Methods in Natural Language Processing, Sydney, Australia, July 2006
41. Russell, J.A., Snodgrass, J.: Emotion and the environment. In: Stokols, D., Altman, I. (eds.) Handbook of Environmental Psychology. Wiley, New York (1987)
42. Sbattella, L.: La Mente Orchestra. Elaborazione della risonanza e autismo, Vita e pensiero (2006)
43. Sbattella, L.: Ti penso, dunque suono. Costrutti cognitivi e relazionali del comportamento musicale: un modello di ricerca-azione. Vita e pensiero (2013)
44. Scherer, K.: What are emotions? and how can they be measured? Soc. Sci. Inf. 44(4), 695–729 (2005)
45. Shi, Y., Song, W.: Speech emotion recognition based on data mining technology. In: Sixth International Conference on Natural Computation (2010)
46. Shriberg, E., Stolcke, A.: Prosody modeling for automatic speech recognition and understanding. In: Proceeding of ISCA Workshop on Prosody in Speech Recognition and Understanding (2001)
47. Shriberg, E., Stolcke, A., Hakkani-Tr, D., Tr, G.: Prosody-based automatic segmentation of speech into sentences and topics. Speech Commun. 32(1–2), 127–154 (2000)
48. Stern, D.: Il mondo interpersonale del bambino, 1st edn. Bollati Boringhieri, Torino (1985)
49. Tesser, F., Cosi, P., Orioli, C., Tisato, G.: Modelli prosodici emotivi per la sintesi dell'italiano. ITC-IRST, ISTC-CNR (2004)
50. Tomkins, S.: Affect theory. In: Sherer, K.R., Ekman, P. (eds.) Approaches to Emotion. Lawrence Erlbaum Associates, Hillsdale (1982)
51. Wang, C., Li, Y.: A study on the search of the most discriminative speech features in the speaker dependent speech emotion recognition. In: International Symposium on Parallel Architectures, Algorithms and Programming (PAAP 2012) (2012)

Multiresolution Feature Extraction During Psychophysiological Inference: Addressing Signals Asynchronicity

François Courtemanche[1](✉), Aude Dufresne[2], and Élise L. LeMoyne[1]

[1] Tech3Lab, HEC Montréal, Louis-Colin av, Montréal, Canada
{francois.courtemanche,elise.labonte-lemoyne}@hec.ca
[2] Department of Communication, University of Montréal,
Édouard-Montpetit blvd, Montréal, Canada
aude.dufresne@umontreal.ca

Abstract. Predicting the psychological state of the user using physiological measures is one of the main objectives of physiological computing. While numerous works have addressed this task with great success, a large number of challenges remain to be solved in order to develop recognition approaches that can precisely and reliably feed human-computer interaction systems. This chapter focuses on one of these challenges which is the temporal asynchrony between different physiological signals within one recognition model. The chapter proposes a flexible and suitable method for feature extraction based on empirical optimisation of windows' latency and duration. The approach is described within the theoretical framework of the psychophysiological inference and its common implementation using machine learning. The method has been experimentally validated (46 subjects) and results are presented. Empirically optimised values for the extraction windows are provided.

Keywords: Affective signal processing · Temporal construction · Psychophysiological inference · Triangulation

1 Introduction

The idea of a link between patterns of physiological activity and psychological states is commonly attributed to the American psychologist William James (1842–1910) [1]. He suggested that a person's perception of emotion stems from physical sensations caused by a reaction to a stimulus. In the early 1990s, computer scientists broadened this idea to create a new field of research: physiological computing [2]. The goal of physiological computing is to translate bioelectrical signals from the human nervous system into computational data. A wide range of applications in human-computer interactions, from brain-computer interactions to affective computing, require the recording and processing of the user's nervous system activity.

This chapter focuses on one subfield of physiological computing that aims to connect physiological measures with psychological states. At a theoretical level, this process is based on the psychophysiological inference [3], and can be defined as follows: let ψ be the set of psychological constructs (e.g. arousal, cognitive load) and Φ

© Springer-Verlag Berlin Heidelberg 2014
H.P. da Silva et al. (Eds.): PhyCS 2014, LNCS 8908, pp. 43–56, 2014.
DOI: 10.1007/978-3-662-45686-6_3

be the set of physiological variables (e.g. heart rate, pupil dilation). [4] now describe the psychophysiological inference according to the following equation:

$$\Psi = f(\Phi) \tag{1}$$

The relationship f could be declined in four ways: (1) one-to-one: a psychological state linked in an isomorphic manner to a physiological variable, (2) one-to-many: a psychological state reflects various physiological variables, (3) many-to-one: various psychological states related to a single physiological variable, or (4) many-to-many: multiple psychological states linked to multiple physiological variables. The regulation of emotions relies at once upon the sympathetic and parasympathetic activity of the autonomic nervous system, whose activity is also integrated in the central nervous system. The regulation of emotion thus requires physiological adjustments stemming from multiple response patterns [5]. Hence, relationships 1 and 3 have little chance of being sufficiently specific to produce a valid inference. In fact, the relationships 2 and 4 dominate the psychophysiology literature. However, when taking into account the difficulties associated with isolating the physiological effects of multiple simultaneous psychological states, most works in physiological computing bring forth the third relationship (many-to-one).

Numerous works have implemented the physiological inference using a machine learning framework [6–12]. Despite interesting results, reported prediction accuracy rates are still below the level of other machine learning problems and cannot feed large-scale real-world applications [13]. In a recent series of papers, [14] proposed 11 prerequisites to strengthen the foundation of this field, which they coined Affective Signal Processing (ASP). In this paper, we specifically address one of these problems; temporal construction [15]. We propose a method to take into account the temporal differences while integrating different physiological signals in a recognition process.

The remainder of the chapter is as follows. Section 2 presents the general inference framework used in this chapter and in most ASP approaches. Section 3 describes the temporal construction problem in the context of the later framework and our approach to address this problem. The experimental validation is presented in Sect. 4 and a discussion and a conclusion are in Sect. 5.

2   Inference Framework

Most works using the psychophysiological inference follow more or less the six steps pipeline summarised in Fig. 1. The main goal is to gather a data set, in which data points have the form $[\Psi_1, \Psi_2, \Psi_3 ..., \Phi]$, in order to train a recognition model f. General definitions of these steps are given is this section and their specific implementations in this work are describe in Sect. 4.

At step 1, the physiological signals Φ_1 are selected according to their relation to the psychological construct Ψ that is to be inferred. In this chapter, three recognition models have been trained to test the temporal construction solution: Ψ_1 = emotional valence, Ψ_2 = emotional arousal and Ψ_3 = cognitive load, and five physiological signals have been selected: Φ_1 = electrodermal activity, Φ_2 = pupil size, Φ_3 = respiration, Φ_4 = electroencephalography, and Φ_5 = cardiovascular activity.

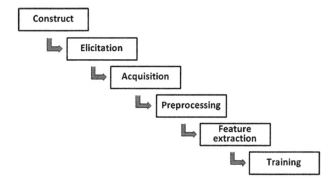

Fig. 1. Psychophysiological inference pipeline

The goal of the elicitation step is to allow subjects to experience different levels of the inferred construct. Elicitation methods can be categorised as being endogenous (relying on voluntary expression) or exogenous (using stimuli) [16]. Whatever the method, the objective it to capture the ground truth (GT) - the real state of the construct for the subject - as precisely as possible. On the other hand, the expected elicitation represents the value that is anticipated and that will be inserted as targets in the training data set (i.e. Φ in a data point). The elicitation error (E_E) can then be defined as $E_E = |GT - \Phi|$. Since GT is related to the experiential dimension of the construct, a certain level of elicitation error is inevitable. As E_E can considerably impair the training process by inducing fuzzy targets, different methods are used to minimise it.

The preprocessing step usually consists in three main sub-steps: denoising, artefact removal and baselining. Denoising aims at removing certain characteristics of the signals generated by the experimental environment, sometimes referred as non-bio-logical artefacts. Most noise sources stem from electrical sources (e.g. outlets, neon, speakers) [17]. The second substep, is intended to remove artefacts from the signals. Artefacts are alterations of the signal due to a subject's movements. Their non-periodic and random nature renders them hard to remove automatically. Therefore, great care needs to be taken to reduce artifacts at the acquisition step (e.g. hand rest, precise instructions, appropriate room temperature). The final substep, baselining is essential in order to compare multiple subjects. Since physiological signals are prone to important interpersonal variations, raw values cannot be used in the inference process [15]. Baselining is then used to correct signals in order to obtain a standard level allowing comparison from different subjects.

The feature extraction step consists of transforming the raw physiological signals in a data representation that will serve as inputs for the training algorithms. The choice of representation can have a significant influence on the training process and it is rec-ommended to use domain knowledge in doing it [18]. In the field of affective signal processing (ASP), most researches use a feature-based approach, popularised by the work of Picard et al. [11]. As illustrated in Fig. 2, this approach consists in three main substeps. First, different underlying features (e.g. Respiratory Sinus Arrhythmia (RSA), heart rate) related to the inferred construct are derived from the raw signal (e.g. Electrocardiogram - ECG). The second substep consists in segmenting these features according to the stimuli presentations. During the last substep, different statistics are calculated over each segment and for each feature (e.g. average, standard deviation, min and max). The latter statistics are the final ψ_i attribute forming a data point.

2.1 Temporal Construction

Finally, an inference model is trained using the resulting data set. This step is composed of two substeps: feature selection and model training. Feature selection consists of selecting an optimal subset of attributes that will be used in model training, and can have different goals: to reduce storage size, to improve the model's performance and to allow a better understanding of data [18]. In the context of the psychophysiological inference, model training consists in using a machine learning algorithms to find the best approximation for the f relationship (see Eq. 1). Many algorithms have been used for this task [19, 20] and there seems to be no a priori best solution. Model performance is assessed using the generalisation error measuring how well the model fit unseen data [21]. Similarly, in the specific context of the psychophysiological inference, genericity represents how well the model fit unseen subjects. There's three main types of models regarding genericity [22]:

1. Subject-dependent: the training set contains data from a single subject and the test set contains new data from the same subject.
2. Subject-independent: the training set contains data from multiple subjects and the test set contains data from new subjects.
3. Mixed dependency: the training set contains data from multiple subjects and the test set contains new data from the same subjects.

Subject independent approaches usually have a higher generalisation error [23] due to individual differences in individual response specificities [24]. However, subject-dependent and mixed approaches have a higher practical value since they don't need to be retrained for each new subject for which they are used. Temporal construction.

Among the 11 prerequisites to improving the field of ASP presented by van den Broek et al. [14], one of the most important is temporal construction. More precisely, three main problems are encountered concerning the temporal aspects of physiological signals [15].

First of all, the habituation phenomenon implies that the intensity of the physiological reactions to the repeated presentation of a stimulus tapers off in time. From the perspective of the psychophysiological inference this means the relationship $\Psi = f(\Phi)$ between a set of signals and a psychological construct is not fixed in time. Other elements must be considered in order to account for the impact of previous occurrences of Ψ upon the physiological reactions at a specific point in time.

The second problem concerns the law of initial values. This law stipulates that "change of any function of an organism due to a stimulus depends, to a large degree, on the prestimulus level of that function" [25]. The use of this law in psychophysiology is subject to debate and it is recommended to discuss the principle of initial values instead [26]. While this principle cannot be applied integrally and should be nuanced, it remains that we can observe a correlation between the prestimulus baseline of a function and the direction and intensity of a reaction.

The final challenge concerning the temporality of physiological activity is the asynchrony of signals. As each physiological system operates in collaboration with a variety of inputs and outputs from the rest of the organism, the measured signals present various durations and latencies for a given stimulus. Heart rate for example may have a shorter latency than Electrodermal Activity (EDA) for a given stimulus. In this context, latency is defined as the time elapsed between the presentation of a stimulus and the beginning of a physiological reaction. Duration is defined as the time elapsed between the start and the end of a physiological reaction. It is harder to identify the end of a reaction as opposed to the beginning because the return to the equilibrium of a signal is not necessarily equivalent to the measured pre-stimulus baseline.

According to [27, 28] and to the best of our knowledge, the current literature on ASP offers no solutions to these three temporal construction problems. We were unable to find methodological approaches or algorithms allowing for the process of inference to take into account these temporal effects and to improve the quality of recognition. Among the three problems, we believe the most critical to be the asynchrony of signals. First, because the relationships 1 and 3 for the psychological inference are not specific enough (see Sect. 1). Second, because signal integration is at the heart of the problem of triangulation of research tools in this field. Asynchrony of signals is thus one of the main obstacles in using multiple physiological signals within a recognition approach. As can be seen in Fig. 2, the feature extraction step segments all the signals at the same time point for a given stimulus. The data vectors forming the training set therefore contain attributes that do not optimally portray the studied construct in regards to latency and duration.

2.2   Windows Optimisation

Our proposed solution for the problem of asynchrony relies upon a flexible feature extraction procedure, which allows modeling of the temporal particularities of the various physiological measures. The main idea is to optimise the latency and duration of extraction windows. As suggested by AlZoubi *et al.* [23], multiresolution extraction windows should lead to better prediction accuracy Furthermore, latency and duration

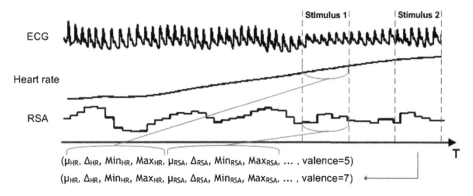

Fig. 2. Feature extraction step

should be optimised according to the different inferred constructs [15]. Consequently, an optimal extraction window should be determined for each attribute and for each construct.

The identification of optimal latencies and durations is done using an empirical optimisation process. This optimisation was performed using the data collected in the experiment described in Sect. 4. Let us take for example the optimisation of the latency of the attribute μ EDA for the construct of emotional arousal. Let n = the number of data points in the training set and L = all possible latencies (e.g. between 0 and 7000 ms, in increments of 100 ms). For each latency L_i, a table of size n × 2 is generated containing n pairs [μ EDA, arousal] using an extraction window with latency L_i. A Pearson correlation coefficient r_i^2 is then computed between both columns of the table. The latency L_i that maximises r_i^2 will be selected as the optimal latency for the feature extraction window of μ EDA for emotional arousal. Figure 3 illustrates various

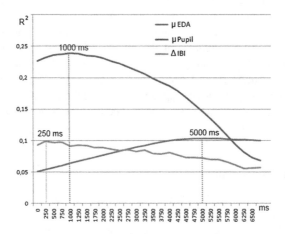

Fig. 3. Empirical optimisation of windows latency

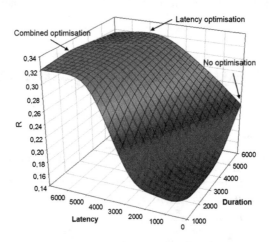

Fig. 4. Combined optimisation of latency and duration

latency values for three attributes (Δ interbeat interval, μ EDA, and μ pupil size), for the construct of emotional arousal. The latencies with the maximal r^2 are identified with dotted lines (5000 ms for μ EDA, 250 ms for Δ IBI (Interbeat Interval), and 1000 ms for μ Pupil).

In order to simultaneously optimise both parameters of the extraction windows, the empirical optimisation process is extended to include duration. As illustrated in Fig. 4 (for μ EDA), for each latency L_i and each duration D_j, a Pearson correlation coefficient r_{ij} is computed.

The previously obtained optimal latency, 5000 ms, goes up to 7000 ms when jointly optimised with duration for μ EDA. This shift on the optimisation surface results in a slight increase of r of 0.01 (0.33–0.32). However, as opposed to the no optimisation point (0, 6000) – stimuli were presented for 6 s (see Sect. 4.1.2) – the impact of the combined optimisation of extraction windows parameters upon r is more substantial (0.33–0.23 = 0.1). The average gain for the correlation coefficients brought on by combined optimisation, for all the attributes of the three inference models, are of 0.08 (arousal), 0.06 (valence) and 0.14 (cognitive load).

3 Validation

This section presents the experimental validation that was performed in order to assess the impact of the optimisation of the feature extraction windows on recognition performance.

3.1 Protocol

Fifty-two (52) participants (average age = 31) were recruited for this experiment, an equal number of men and women. A compensation of 40$ was offered at the end of the session, which lasted about 1h30.

The physiological signals were collected at 250 Hz using a Procomp Inifinity amplifier from Thought Technology. Electrodermal activity (EDA) was recorded at the phalange site. Cardiovascular activity was recorded through blood volume pressure (BVP) using a photopletismograph placed on the middle finger. A respiration belt placed on the upper chest was used to record respiration activity. Electroencephalographic (EEG) activity was recorded using four electrodes on the F3, F4, P3 and P4 sites following the 10–20 placement system. These sites were selected in order to measure frontal asymmetry [29]. A 60 Hz notch filter, and low-pass (1 Hz) and high-pass (60 Hz) filter were applied to remove the electrical noise. Finally, pupil size was measured using a Tobii X-120 eye-tracker. A simple normalisation procedure was applied ($x' = x - \mu B$) using baseline data collected during a two-minute resting period before acquisition.

For this work, 20 features were extracted from the resulting preprocessed signals using the method described in Sect. 2, for which 7 statistics were calculated (mean, standard deviation, average and absolute values of the first difference, min, max, and kurtosis). Each data point in the training set is initially composed of 140 attributes and one target.

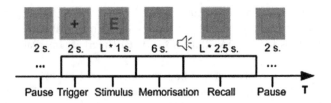

Fig. 5. Cognitive load stimuli presentation sequence

Cognitive load elicitation. The first 15 participants did not complete the cognitive load task. Amongst the 37 participants that completed this part of the experiment, data from six was rejected because of technical problems related to the recording of physiological signals. Hence, data from 31 participants was retained.

The protocol used to elicit cognitive load consisted of an immediate serial recall task. Twenty-four sequences of letters, varying between two and seven letters, were presented to the participants. They were asked to retain them for six seconds, before repeating them out loud. The first 12 sequences were repeated in the same order they were presented, while the following 12 were repeated in the inverse order. The memorising was solely mental and repeated voicing strategies were prohibited. The presentation sequence of the stimuli is shown in Fig. 5.

The beginning of the sequence was indicated by the presence of a green cross. Then followed the sequence of letters, each presented for one second, and the period of memorising. An audible beep signaled when the presented sequence should be repeated. This task provided 744 training examples.

Arousal and valence elicitation. Standardised stimuli composed of an image and a related sound from the International Affective Picture System (IAPS) [30] and the International Affective Digitized Sounds (IADS) [31] collections were used to elicit emotional arousal and valence. Forty-six stimuli were presented for a period of six seconds each. A bimodal stimuli approach was chosen in order to confer a stronger ecological validity to the elicitation [32, 33]. Self-evaluation using the SAM scale [34] has also been used in order to reduce the elicitation error (see Sect. 2).

All participants performed the affective stimuli task. Data from eight of them were rejected because of technical problems tied to the recording of physiological signals. Hence, data from 44 participants was retained. While relying upon the normalised evaluation of the valence and arousal of the stimuli included in the IAPS, the images were chosen in order to form five groups and uniformly cover all quadrants of the emotional space. Figure 6 shows the distribution of the selected images.

The distribution includes four non neutral groups composed of eight images each: negative/low, negative/high, positive/low and positive/high, as well as a neutral group composed of 14 images: neutral/very low. The sequence of the affective stimuli presentations is depicted in Fig. 7.

The general sequence, at the top of the figure, alternates neutral and non-neutral block with a 20 s break in between each. The neutral and non-neutral blocks respectively include two and four stimuli. The bottom of the figure shows the sequence of presentations within a block. It begins with a baseline (2 s), followed by the presentation of a

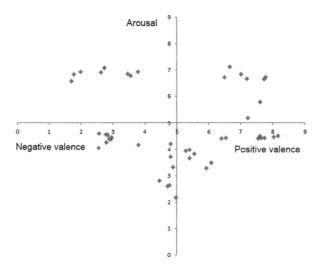

Fig. 6. Affective distribution of stimuli

stimulus (6 s) and ends with a rest period (5 s). The presentation order of the non-neutral blocks and the presentation order of the images inside of the blocks are random. The images were presented full screen and a green cross was displayed for one second before each image. After all 46 stimuli were presented, a self-assessment interface was introduced showing all the previously shown images in the same order. Underneath each image were two scales based upon the Self-Assessment Manikin (SAM) allowing for the rating of the emotion felt at the time of the original presentation. They were scored on a scale of 1–9. This task produced 2024 training examples.

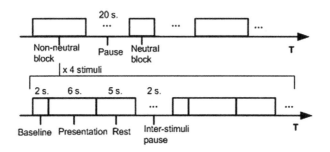

Fig. 7. Affective stimuli presentation sequence

3.2   Results

Prior to model training, a substep of feature selection was performed in order to reduce the data dimensionality and to keep only the more relevant attributes. A variable ranking method based on random probes was used [18], and 38 physiological attributes were selected for the arousal model, 10 for the valence model and 51 for the cognitive load model. For emotional arousal and valence, the targets are the average between the subject's self-assessment and the normalised values from the IAPS and IADS guides. For the cognitive load model, the targets are the number of letters to memorise (2–7). Since all targets are numbers, the training of each model is a regression problem. As we are interested in assessing the impact of the proposed temporal construction method on recognition performance (and not recognition performance per se), three different training algorithms were used: Support Machine Vectors (SVM), k-Nearest Neighbor (KNN) and Artificial Neural Networks (ANN). The Statistica software from Statsoft was used to perform training.

For machine learning regression problem, the quality of the model's training is assessed using the mean squared error (MSE), which is the average of the squared difference between the predictions and the actual values. Results are presented according to this metric. Training of the SVM and KNN models was executed following a k-fold cross validation procedure with k = 10. Training of the ANN model was executed 10 times and the results averaged out to account for the randomised elements involved in the training procedure. In order to assess the impact of temporal construction method upon the capacity of the models to recognise the emotional/cognitive state of a subject, the models were trained with and without extraction windows optimisation. Results are presented in Fig. 8.

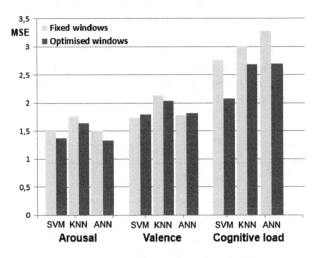

Fig. 8. Impact of windows optimisation on MSE

We can see that the mean squared error (MSE) variation trends for each construct were consistent amongst the different algorithms except for emotional valence where two algorithms (SVM and ANN) suffered a small error increase while one algorithm decreased (KNN). The average variation of MSE (over the three algorithms) for each model is of −0.15 (arousal), 0.0 (valence) and −0.53 (cognitive load). This results in average proportional gains for the prediction performance of 9 % (arousal), 0 % (valence) and 18 % (cognitive load).

4   Discussion/Conclusion

van den Broek et al. proposed 11 prerequisites to strengthen the foundation of affective signal processing [14]. This chapter presented a solution to the specific problem of signal asynchrony. We demonstrated a method to circumvent the temporal differences while integrating many different signals in an implementation of the psychophysiological inference $\Psi = f(\Phi)$. When the relationship f is used on a one-to-many basis (a psychological state reflects various physiological variables), the elements of Φ react according to different temporal scales (e.g. EDA at 4 s and ECG at 1 s post stimulus). Until now, the feature extraction methods used in the literature neglected this phenomenon and segmented all signals according to a stimulus using a single window.

Our temporal construction technique provides a solution to the problem of signal asynchrony and allows for a more optimal triangulation of multiple signals and recording instruments by individually optimising each extraction window for both latency and duration. Results from this experiment showed how the technique improved the quality of recognition model of arousal by 9 % and of cognitive load by 18 %. The valence recognition model was not improved (0 %) on the average and reduced for two algorithms (SVM and ANN). A possible explanation for this can be found in the bipolar nature of the valence scale. As opposed to arousal and cognitive load which increase in a monotonous way, valence can be conceived as evolving in two directions (positive or negative). Indeed, it has been suggested to replace the bipolar scale with two unipolar scales [35]. With this in mind it is logical that a unique relationship between values from the bipolar scale and optimal temporal windows is hard to establish. We now believe that different optimal windows can exist for a given physiological signal, depending upon the positivity or negativity of valence. Future works should also include looking for gender, age or personality effects on the value of the optimal windows' latency and duration. It could therefore be possible to tailor more precisely the extraction windows for specific subjects.

Following the large sample size of this study (n = 44 for valence and arousal and n = 31 for cognitive load), it can be expected that the empirically optimised values for the extraction windows can be used successfully in other studies. To do so, we included in the Appendix (Fig. 9) the aforementioned values. Researchers working on the physiological recognition of valence, arousal or cognitive load could use these values while segmenting signals according to their stimuli – being that they are alike – and look for a gain in recognition accuracy. The proposed approach could also be adapted to different recognition contexts by optimising extraction windows for various physiological signals, psychological constructs or stimuli.

Acknowledgements. This work was supported by NSERC (Natural Sciences and Engineering Research Council of Canada), the Canadian Space Agency and Bell Canada. The authors would like to thank the Bell Web Solutions User Experience Center for providing the eye-tracker system used in this research. We also wish to thank Laurence Dumont for early comments on the manuscript.

Appendix

Left table:

Signal	Feature	Attribute	Arousal L	Arousal D	Valence L	Valence D	CL L	CL D
BVP	Heart rate	μ	0	1000	4750	1000	0	2600
		std	0	5750	0	1000	2200	1000
		μΔ	3000	1250	2750	2750	5800	3600
		|Δ|	750	4250	0	1000	2200	1000
		min	1000	1250	3000	2750	0	1400
		max	0	5750	6250	1250	7000	3600
		kurtosis	4750	5500	3500	2500	2200	5800
	Interbeat interval (IBI)	μ	7000	2250	0	1000	400	5600
		std	250	6000	6250	1250	2200	1000
		μΔ	4250	4750	5500	5500	2400	5400
		|Δ|	500	5750	0	1000	2200	1800
		min	7000	1000	0	1000	4000	4600
		max	7000	4000	0	1000	1000	1600
		kurtosis	4750	5500	3500	2500	2200	5600
	Amplitude	μ	0	1000	0	1000	5400	1600
		std	2750	5750	0	1000	1800	1600
		μΔ	1000	2750	3750	2750	5000	1600
		|Δ|	5750	2000	0	1000	2000	1200
		min	0	1000	0	1000	5200	1000
		max	2750	5500	0	1000	3800	1400
		kurtosis	4250	5000	4000	3000	5800	4800
	VLF (% of total power)	μ	0	1000	0	1000	0	1000
		std	6250	2250	0	1000	0	1200
		μΔ	6000	1250	7000	1750	0	1000
		|Δ|	6750	1500	0	1000	0	1200
		min	0	1000	0	1000	0	1000
		max	0	1000	0	1000	0	1000
		kurtosis	0	1500	6750	1250	0	3800
	LF (% of total power)	μ	7000	6000	0	1000	0	1200
		std	0	1000	0	1000	200	1000
		μΔ	7000	2250	0	1000	0	1000
		|Δ|	0	1250	0	1000	200	1000
		min	7000	6000	0	1000	0	1200
		max	7000	6000	0	1000	0	1400
		kurtosis	0	1500	5750	4500	3400	1000
	HF (% of total power)	μ	3750	1000	0	1000	0	1000
		std	0	1000	0	1000	0	1000
		μΔ	0	1000	0	1000	0	1000
		|Δ|	0	1000	0	1000	0	1000
		min	0	5250	0	1000	0	1000
		max	6000	6000	0	1000	0	1000
		kurtosis	6250	1000	6500	1500	800	1200
	LF/HF (% of total power)	μ	7000	6000	0	1000	0	1200
		std	2750	4750	0	1000	3800	1000
		μΔ	0	1000	0	1000	0	1000
		|Δ|	4250	2250	0	1000	2800	1000
		min	7000	6000	0	1000	0	1200
		max	7000	6000	0	1000	0	1200
		kurtosis	3250	1250	6500	1750	7000	2800
	VLF (average power)	μ	0	1000	7000	6000	7000	6000
		std	5750	3500	1000	1000	0	1000
		μΔ	6500	1250	0	1000	0	1000
		|Δ|	5500	4250	1000	1000	0	1000
		min	0	1000	3500	6000	7000	5000
		max	0	1000	1000	1000	7000	6000
		kurtosis	1000	1750	3250	1250	1200	1200
	LF (average power)	μ	0	1000	0	1000	0	1000
		std	0	1000	4250	1250	0	1000
		μΔ	0	1000	0	1000	0	1000
		|Δ|	0	1000	3750	2750	0	1000
		min	0	1000	0	3000	0	1000
		max	0	1000	0	1000	0	1000
		kurtosis	3750	2000	500	3500	4800	1000
	HF (average power)	μ	1500	6000	0	1000	0	5600
		std	7000	6000	0	1000	1600	4800
		μΔ	0	1000	0	1000	6800	1000
		|Δ|	7000	6000	0	1000	2000	3800
		min	3000	1000	0	1000	1000	2400
		max	7000	6000	0	1000	2400	1400
		kurtosis	7000	6000	250	3250	400	1400

Right table:

Signal	Feature	Attribute	Arousal L	Arousal D	Valence L	Valence D	CL L	CL D
BVP	LF/HF (average power)	μ	7000	6000	0	1000	0	1200
		std	2750	4750	0	1000	3800	1000
		μΔ	0	1000	0	1000	0	1000
		|Δ|	5000	1250	0	1000	3800	1000
		min	7000	6000	0	1000	200	1000
		max	7000	6000	0	1000	0	1200
		kurtosis	6750	1750	0	2250	6200	1600
	HR Max-Min	μ	3000	6000	0	1000	0	1000
		std	4500	3000	1000	1000	0	1000
		μΔ	1000	1500	7000	3750	2800	5800
		|Δ|	4500	2750	750	1000	0	1000
		min	3750	1250	0	1000	6800	1400
		max	2500	4750	0	1000	6000	5000
		kurtosis	6750	3500	6500	6000	6000	4800
EDA	Skin conductance	μ	7000	2750	0	1000	7000	6000
		std	3500	2000	0	1000	7000	6000
		μΔ	3250	2000	6500	5500	6600	6000
		|Δ|	3750	1500	0	1000	6600	6000
		min	7000	2250	0	1000	7000	4000
		max	5500	4250	0	1000	7000	6000
		kurtosis	0	5000	0	1000	2400	1200
EEG	F3-F4	μ	0	1000	0	1000	0	1000
		std	1000	1500	1500	1000	5400	3800
		μΔ	3250	5750	3500	3500	5200	1000
		|Δ|	1250	1500	0	2250	4400	5800
		min	0	1000	0	1000	0	1000
		max	7000	4750	1500	1000	6800	5800
		kurtosis	2500	2250	5500	1250	1200	4200
	P3-P4	μ	500	1750	0	1000	0	1000
		std	0	1000	0	1000	3800	1000
		μΔ	0	3250	7000	2250	3400	1000
		|Δ|	5750	2000	0	1000	2000	1200
		min	0	1000	0	1000	5200	1000
		max	2750	5500	0	1000	3800	1400
		kurtosis	4250	5000	4000	3000	5800	4800
	(F3+P3) - (F4+P4)	μ	750	2250	0	1000	0	1000
		std	0	1250	7000	6000	3800	1000
		μΔ	1000	3750	3500	5750	1400	1000
		|Δ|	1500	1000	0	1000	4000	2000
		min	750	2500	0	1000	0	1000
		max	250	1500	0	1000	4600	4000
		kurtosis	2750	1750	4250	2750	0	2200
	(F3+F4) - (P3+P4)	μ	3750	1000	6500	1000	2000	6000
		std	7000	6000	0	1000	6600	5000
		μΔ	1750	2500	2000	5250	0	2600
		|Δ|	6750	3750	0	1000	7000	5200
		min	3250	1500	7000	2250	2600	1000
		max	2250	2500	6500	1000	2200	2600
		kurtosis	2500	1250	5500	1750	800	2200
Resp.	Respiration rate	μ	3000	1000	0	1000	0	1000
		std	750	1000	0	1000	1400	2000
		μΔ	0	1000	5750	1000	0	1000
		|Δ|	750	1000	750	1500	1600	1600
		min	1750	1750	0	1000	0	1000
		max	3500	1250	6500	5000	0	3200
		kurtosis	2500	3500	6500	1500	5400	5200
	Amplitude	μ	5500	3500	0	1000	0	1000
		std	2750	1250	0	1000	7000	5000
		μΔ	0	1000	1500	3250	2000	3600
		|Δ|	2750	1000	0	1000	0	1000
		min	1500	3750	0	1000	0	1000
		max	5000	3000	0	1000	3000	1400
		kurtosis	2500	3500	6500	6000	4800	5600
Pupil	Size	μ	4500	1000	7000	2000	7000	3200
		std	0	2000	7000	3750	4600	1400
		μΔ	500	1000	3000	4500	800	2800
		|Δ|	4750	2500	4750	1000	4000	1400
		min	4500	1000	7000	5500	7000	2400
		max	5000	1750	7000	1250	7000	5200
		kurtosis	1500	5250	2750	6000	5000	6000

References

1. Ellsworth, P.C.: William James and emotion: Is a century of fame worth a century of misunderstanding? Psychol. Rev. **101**(2), 222–229 (1994)
2. Allanson, J., Fairclough, S.H.: A research agenda for physiological computing. Interact. Comput. **16**(5), 857–878 (2004)
3. Cacioppo, J.T., Tassinary, L.G.: Inferring psychological significance from physiological signals. Am. Psychol. **45**(1), 16–28 (1990)

4. Cacioppo, J.T., Tassinary, L.T., Berntson, G., et al.: Psychophysiological science: interdisciplinary approaches to classic questions about the mind. In: Cacioppo, J.T., Tassinary, L.G., Berntson, G. (eds.) Handbook of Psychophysiology, pp. 1–18. Cambride University Press, New York (2007)
5. Kreibig, S.D.: Autonomic nervous system activity in emotion: a review. Biol. Psychol. **84** (3), 394–421 (2010)
6. Bamidis, P., et al.: An integrated approach to emotion recognition for advanced emotional intelligence. In: Jacko, J. (ed.) Human-Computer Interaction. Ambient, Ubiquitous and Intelligent Interaction, pp. 565–574. Springer, Berlin (2009)
7. Chanel, G., et al.: Short-term emotion assessment in a recall paradigm. Int. J. Hum Comput Stud. **67**(8), 607–627 (2009)
8. Christie, I.C., Friedman, B.H.: Autonomic specificity of discrete emotion and dimensions of affective space: a multivariate approach. Int. J. Psychophysiol. **51**(2), 143–153 (2004)
9. Haag, A., Goronzy, S., Schaich, P., Williams, J.: Emotion recognition using bio-sensors: first steps towards an automatic system. In: André, E., Dybkjær, L., Minker, W., Heisterkamp, P. (eds.) ADS 2004. LNCS (LNAI), vol. 3068, pp. 36–48. Springer, Heidelberg (2004)
10. Kolodyazhniy, V., et al.: An affective computing approach to physiological emotion specificity: toward subject-independent and stimulus-independent classification of film-induced emotions. Psychophysiology **48**(7), 908–922 (2011)
11. Picard, R.W., Vyzas, E., Healey, J.: Toward machine emotional intelligence: analysis of affective physiological state. IEEE Trans. Pattern Anal. Mach. Intell. **23**(10), 1175 (2001)
12. Verhoef, T., et al.: Bio-sensing for emotional characterization without word labels. In: Jacko, J. (ed.) Human-Computer Interaction. Ambient, Ubiquitous and Intelligent Interaction, pp. 693–702. Springer, Berlin (2009)
13. van den Broek, E., et al.: Prerequisites for affective signal processing (ASP) - Part III. In: Third International Conference on Bio-Inspired Systems and Signal Processing, Biosignals 2010. Valencia, Spain (2010)
14. van den Broek, E., et al.: Prerequisites for affective signal processing (ASP). In: International Conference on Bio-inspired Systems and Signal Processing. INSTICC Press, Portugal (2009)
15. van den Broek, E., et al.: Prerequisites for affective signal processing (ASP) - Part IV. In: 1st International Workshop on Bio-Inspired Human-Machine Interfaces and Healthcare Applications - B-Interface 2010, pp. 59–66. Valencia, Spain 2010
16. Cowie, R., et al.: Issues in data collection. In: Cowie, R., Pelachaud, C., Petta, P. (eds.) Emotion-Oriented Systems, pp. 197–212. Springer, Berlin (2011)
17. Pizzagalli, D.A., et al.: Electoencephalography and high-density electrophysiological source localisation. In: Cacioppo, J.T., Tassinary, L.G., Bernston, G.G. (eds.) Handbook of Psychophysiology, pp. 56–84. Cambride University Press, New York (2007)
18. Guyon, I., Elisseeff, A.: An introduction to variable and feature selection. J. Mach. Learn. Res. **3**, 1157–1182 (2003)
19. Rani, P., et al.: An empirical study of machine learning techniques for affect recognition in human–robot interaction. Pattern Anal. Appl. **9**(1), 58–69 (2006)
20. Zhihong, Z., et al.: A survey of affect recognition methods: audio, visual, and spontaneous expressions. IEEE Trans. Pattern Anal. Mach. Intell. **31**(1), 39–58 (2009)
21. Bishop, C.M.: Pattern Recognition and Machine Learning. Springer, New York (2006)
22. Kim, J., Elesabeth, A., Thurid, V.: Towards user-independent classification of multimodal emotional signals. In: 3rd International Conference on Affective Computing and Intelligent Interaction and Workshops (ACII 2009) (2009)

23. AlZoubi, O., D'Mello, S.K., Calvo, R.A.: Detecting naturalistic expressions of nonbasic affect using physiological signals. IEEE Trans. Affect. Comput. **3**(3), 298–310 (2012)

24. Schuster, T., et al.: EEG-based valence recognition: what do we know about the influence of individual specificity? In: The Fourth International Conference on Advanced Cognitive Technologies and Applications (COGNITIVE 2012). Nice, France (2012)

25. Wilder, J.: Modern psychophysiology and the law of initial value. Am. J. Psychother. **12**, 199–221 (1958)

26. Jennings, L.R., Gianaros, P.J., et al.: Methodology. In: Cacioppo, J.T., Tassinary, L.G., Bernston, G.G. (eds.) Handbook of Psychophysiology, pp. 812–833. Cambride University Press, New York (2007)

27. Gunes, H., Pantic, M.: Automatic Measurement of Affect in Dimensional and Continuous Spaces: Why, What, and How?. In: Spink, A.J., et al. (eds.) 7th International Conference on Methods and Techniques in Behavioral Research, Measuring Behavior 2010, pp. 122–126. Noldus, Eindhoven (2010)

28. van der Zwaag, M.D., van den Broek, E., Janssen, J.H.: Guidelines for biosignal driven HCI. In: ACM CHI2010 workshop - Brain, Body, and Bytes: Physiological User Interaction. Atlanta, GA, USA (2010)

29. Coan, J.A., Allen, J.J.B.: Frontal EEG asymmetry as a moderator and mediator of emotion. Biol. Psychol. **67**(1–2), 7–50 (2004)

30. Lang, P.J., Bradley, M.M., Cuthbert, B.N: International affective picture system (IAPS): Affective ratings of pictures and instruction manual. Technical report B-3. 2008, University of Florida, Gainesville, FI (2008)

31. Bradley, M.M., Lang, P.J.: The International Affective Digitized Sounds (2nd edn., IADS-2): Affective Ratings of Sounds and Instruction Manual. Technical report B-3, University of Florida, Gainesville, FI (2007)

32. Anttonen, J., Surakka, V.: Emotions and heart rate while sitting on a chair. In: SIGCHI Conference on Human Factors in Computing Systems, pp. 491–499. ACM, Portland (2005)

33. Mühl, C., Heylen, D.: Cross-modal elicitation of affective experience. In: International Conference on Affective Computing and Intelligent Interaction and Workshops (ACII 2009). Workshop on Affective Brain-Computer Interfaces. Amsterdam, The Netherlands (2009)

34. Bradley, M.M., Lang, P.J.: Measuring emotion: The self-assessment manikin and the semantic differential. J. Behav. Ther. Exp. Psychiatry **25**(1), 49–59 (1994)

35. van den Broek, E.: Ubiquitous emotion-aware computing. Pers. Ubiquit. Comput. **17**, 1–15 (2011)

Devices

Paper-Based Inkjet Electrodes
Experimental Study for ECG Applications

Ana Priscila Alves[1]($\boxtimes$), João Martins[2], Hugo Plácido da Silva[1],
André Lourenço[1,3], Ana Fred[1], and Hugo Ferreira[2]

[1] Instituto de Telecomunicações, Instituto Superior Técnico,
Avenida Rovisco Pais, 1, 1049-001 Lisboa, Portugal
{anapriscila.alves,hsilva,arlourenco,afred}@lx.it.pt
[2] Faculdade de Ciências da Universidade de Lisboa,
Alameda da Universidade, 1649-004 Lisbon, Portugal
joaopedr.martins@gmail.com
[3] Instituto Superior de Engenharia de Lisboa,
Rua Conselheiro Emídio Navarro, 1, 1959-007 Lisboa, Portugal
hhferreira@fc.ul.pt

Abstract. Electrocardiographic (ECG) acquisition has evolved imensly
over the last decade in particular with regards to sensing technology.
From classical silver/silver chloride (Ag/AgCl) electrodes, to textile electrodes, and recently paper-based electrodes. In this paper we study a
new type of silver/silver chloride (Ag/AgCl) electrodes based on a paper
substrate that are produced using an inkjet printing technique. The cost
reduction, easy-to-produce methodology, and easier recycling increase
the potencial of application of these electrodes and opens this technology
for everyday life use. We performed a comparison between this new type
of electrode, with classical gelled Ag/AgCl electrodes and dry Ag/AgCl
electrodes. We also compared the performance of each electrode when
acquired using a professional-grade gold standard device, and a low cost
platform. Experimental results showed that data acquired using our proposed inkjet printed electrode is highly correlated with data obtained
through conventional electrodes. Moreover, the electrodes are robust to
both high-end and low-end data acquisition devices.

Keywords: Electrodes · Paper · Inkjet · Electrocardiography · Device

1 Introduction

Electrocardiographic (ECG) signals are probably the most well-known biosignals, and can be found in multiple applications in the medical and quality of
life domains. This signal is commonly used to assess the overall cardiac function, measure the rate and regularity of heartbeats, and detect the presence
of any pathology in the heart. The classical acquisition methods used in clinical or research studies typically recur to gelled silver/silver chloride (Ag/AgCl)
electrodes.

© Springer-Verlag Berlin Heidelberg 2014
H.P. da Silva et al. (Eds.): PhyCS 2014, LNCS 8908, pp. 59–70, 2014.
DOI: 10.1007/978-3-662-45686-6_4

The introduction of new types of electrodes opens the door to a new type of applications, as the acquisition of ECG becames less expensive and more pervasive [1–4].

Paper has several advantages for ECG data acquisition in daily life scenarios; it enables: (a) lower production costs; (b) easier recycling; and (c) simpler production, especially when considering the possibility of inkjet printing. When compared to plastic substrates such as polyethylene terephtalate (PET, ≈ 2 cent dm^{-2}) and polymide (PI, ≈ 30 cent dm^{-2}), paper has significantly lower production costs (≈ 0.1 cent dm^{-2}). In addition to this, considering the active disassembly design principles [5], paper is a good choice due to its environmentally friendly characteristics. Recently, it has been considered as a potential substrate for low-cost flexible electronics [6,7], which motivated us to do research on the possibility of using paper-based electrodes for biosignals acquisition. With such an approach and its ready availability, the electrodes can even be produced by the user himself or his caregivers.

The deposition of the conductive part of the electrodes to the paper substrate can be made recurring to photo-lithography, vacuum processes or printing techniques. The use of printing techniques for fabricating electronics has several advantages over laboratory scale and subtractive batch processes [8]; printing is fast, low-cost, and widely used. In particular digital inkjet printing, which has been used as a research tool, is facilitating initial explorations of various aspects of printed electronics targeting the consumer market [9]. The focus of this work was to explore the potential use of paper-based inkjet printed electrodes for ECG signal acquisition.

The most commonly used type of electrode is the gelled Ag/AgCl electrode; however, to make an acquisition setup more convenient for everyday use applications, other alternatives are emerging. Previous work from our group has started to explore the use of dry Ag/AgCl electrodes [1], which usually leads to signals with lower signal-to-noise ratio, although still suitable for monitoring or other non-intrusive applications. Thus, to study the characteristics of the paper-based inkjet printed electrodes, we performed a comparative study against the most common alternatives: (i) gelled; (ii) dry.

The remainder of the paper is organized as follows: in Sect. 2 we describe the proposed electrodes, focusing on their production and main characteristics; Sects. 3 and 4 present the methodology applied in the comparison of the different electrode types and their quantitative evaluation; and finally, in Sects. 5 and 6 we provide a summary of the experimental results and outline the main conclusions.

2   Paper-Based Inkjet Printed Electrodes

The possibility of printing materials using inkjet technology brought several advantages over the conventional manufacturing procedures used, such as photo-lithography, transfer printing, among others. Comparing with those standard techniques for patterning thin films with high precision, some differences stand out. The appeal of inkjet technology lies in the fact that it is based on contactless deposition, which implies a lesser risk of contaminating the material, it is a mask-less approach that makes an intuitive procedure, and it is an additive procedure, i.e., it is possible to print over a previously printed pattern [9].

Producing electrodes by inkjet printing enables the use of thin and flexible sub-strates that may also be biocompatible, examples of which are polydimethylsilox-ane (PDMS) or biocellulose. On the other hand, low-cost paper-like substrates such as photo paper can be used as an alternative substrate and several conduc-tive inks can already be used, such as silver, gold or conductive polymer [10]).

We fabricated the electrodes using photo paper as substrate, due to its flex-ibility, availability, reduced thickness ($230\,\mu m$) and easy maneuverability. To create the conductive part of the electrode we used a commercial printable sil-ver ink from SunTronic, which is composed of silver nanoparticles and has been shown to provide good electrical conductivity for electronic applications.

The electrodes devised in the scope of our work were designed as a flat rec-tangular shape, with dimensions of $8\,cm$ length, $3\,cm$ width and approximately $1\,\mu m$ thick. Each electrode has a total of $24\,cm^2$ of area in contact with the skin. The electrodes were first printed with four silver layers and afterwards subjected to heat treatment during $20\,min$ at a temperature of $85\,°C$. With this heat treatment, we obtained a silver resistivity of $1.68 \times 10^{-6}\Omega$.

The second step of the fabrication process was to produce a layer which enables the transduction of ionic concentrations measured by electrodes into electrical potentials. At the skin-electrode interface, the ionic signal (Cl^- ion transports the charge) is transformed into an electric signal. Likewise, in common silver electrodes this layer is typically made of AgCl [11]. The formation of this layer was achieved by adding Cl^- ions, enabling a reaction between Ag and Cl to produce AgCl. However, due to the thin layer of silver and the fragility of the photo paper, the amount and the manner of introducing Cl^- ions is important. This process was optimized by using commercial bleach deposited by an airbrush at a distance of approximately $30\,cm$.

The third step in the production of these electrodes was focused on ensuring a good, long lasting, and practical contact between the electrodes and the acqui-sition hardware. To facilitate the connection of cables and make the electrodes practical for regular use, we use a metal stud and conductive snap. The snaps were placed in the back of the printed surface and the communication to the front was made through a hole filled with a conductive silver paste from Agar Scientific.

3   Methodology

We benchmarked the performance of our paper-based inkjet printed electrodes for ECG data acquisition, comparing them both to standard pre-gelled Ag/AgCl electrodes, and to the dry electrodes approach that we have been recently fol-lowing [1]. Reference data was collected using a BIOPAC biosignal acquisition unit, which has seen extensive use in the research domain and is considered to be a gold standard in biomedical research. However, this system has restricted

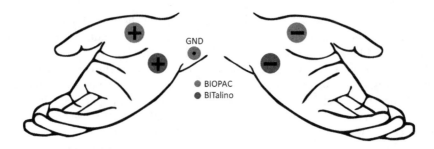

Fig. 1. Electrode placement

operations and experimenting new customized solutions can damage the device. As such, we have used a BITalino acquisition system [12,13], which give us an higher control over the system to try different experimental setups.

This work is aligned with our research towards off-the-person ECG sensing [2], reason for which the ECG signals were acquired in the palmar region of the left and right hands, as illustrated in Fig. 1. The electrodes used for data acquisition with the BIOPAC were always the pre-gelled Ag/AgCl, while with the BITalino we tested the previously mentioned 3 types of electrodes.

We devised our comparative study with two objectives:

1. comparison of the BITalino performance with a gold standard acquisition system, the BIOPAC;
2. comparison of electrodes for ECG acquisition.

The BITalino acquisition device adopts the 2-electrode approach with a virtual ground, while the BIOPAC system is designed to collect data with an additional ground electrode. In order to assess the BIOPAC performance after removing the ground electrode, we performed two experiments: with and without the ground electrode. To evaluate the performance of the dry, and paper-based inkjet electrodes in the ECG acquisition, we did 2 experiments in which we compared them with the pre-gelled ones. The experiments are summarized in Table 1.

Table 1. Summary of the experiments: Type refers to the type of electrodes used; the GND columns indicate if a ground electrode was used (three electrodes in total) or a virtual ground was produced internally (only two electrodes).

Experiment	BIOPAC		BITalino	
	Type	GND	Type	GND
1	Gel	Yes	Gel	No
2	Gel	No	Gel	No
3	Gel	No	Dry	No
4	Gel	No	Paper	No

Each experiment consisted of a 30 s recording performed simultaneously with the BIOPAC and the BITalino; we used a sampling rate of 1000 Hz in both devices and a 12-bit resolution for the BIOPAC, whereas the BITalino has a 10-bit resolution. The BIOPAC raw data was reduced to 10 bits, to be at the same resolution as the BITalino signals. We have collected raw ECG data from 20 subjects in a static standing position, with the electrodes applied as shown in Fig. 1.

The data obtained by each device was pre-processed in three main steps, as represented in Fig. 2.

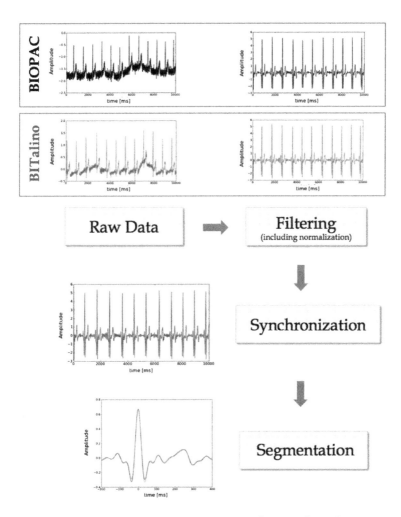

Fig. 2. Block diagram of the pre-processing steps we have performed, to compare the signals acquired from both devices. The curves plotted in black were acquired using the BIOPAC while the blue ones with the BITalino (Color figure online)

Taking the raw data as input, the baseline wander was corrected through a two-stage median filter, as proposed by [14], and the signals were filtered using a Finite Impulse Response (FIR) bandpass filter with a Hamming window of 300 ms, and cutoff frequencies of 5–20 Hz. The filtered signals were normalized to their maximum and minimum amplitudes, where the original signal is subtracted of its mean, and divided by its standard deviation.

To prevent any possible electrical interference between the devices prone to bias the results and resulting from a hard wired connection between both devices, we chose to do the synchronization using the RR time intervals. Given that the comparison of the ECG data obtained from two independent systems can only be correctly performed for data expressed in the same time base, our synchronization method consisted on the following steps:

1. Detection of the QRS complex in each independent signal, using the method proposed by [15].
2. Let $RR_{BIOPAC} = \{RR_{BIOPAC_0}, ..., RR_{BIOPAC_n}\}$ and $RR_{BITalino} = \{RR_{BITalino_0}, ..., RR_{BITalino_m}\}$ be a set of RR time intervals for the n and m heartbeat waveforms detected respectively in the BIOPAC and BITalino ECG time series.
3. Construct a matching matrix, M, in which the entry $M(i, j)$ corresponds to the absolute value of the difference between the RR time intervals extracted from the BIOPAC and BITalino ECG time series, that is:

$$M(i, j) = |RR_{BITalino_i} - RR_{BIOPAC_j}| \qquad (1)$$

4. Let $\#M$ be the number of items where $M(i, j) \leq RR_{th}$.
5. If $\#M > Sync_{th}$, the synchronization is complete. Otherwise, go to next step.
6. Consider $RR_{BITalino}(k) = \{RR_{BITalino_k}, ..., RR_{BITalino_m}\}$. Repeat steps 3 and 4 for each value of $k \in \{1, ..., m\}$ and compute each value of $M(i, j) = |RR_{BITalino_i}(k) - RR_{BIOPAC_j}|$.
7. Find the k value where $\#M$ is higher.
8. Synchronize the signals by applying a delay of k samples to the BITalino signal.

The acquisition was always initiated first with the BITalino, so it has the longer time series. We defined 2 thresholds in the synchronization method, $Sync_{th}$ and RR_{th}. The $Sync_{th}$ value applied was 20, since it is approximately the minimum number of heartbeats expected in a 30 s ECG signal. The RR_{th} threshold represents the minimum difference of RR time intervals, from different acquisitions, where the R peaks are considered to match in the time domain. Since the acquisitions were performed by two different systems, it is expected a small deviation between the instants where the same R peaks occur. Therefore, we considered that 5 ms is the maximum value where the R peaks are considered to occur at the same instant. Finally, the individual heartbeat waveforms were segmented and scaled between 0 and 1; we consider the heartbeat waveform to be the $[-200; 400]$ ms interval centered at the R peak instant.

4   Evaluation Metrics

Two metrics were employed for numerical evaluation purposes, namely the Signal-to-Noise Ratio (SNR) computed from the data collected with both devices for each of the 4 experiments, and the Root Mean Square Error (RMSE) of the cosine distance, to assess the morphological correlation between the heartbeat waveforms obtained with the BIOPAC and the BITalino, when using each type of electrodes. For the SNR calculation, we considered the signal of interest to be concentrated on the 5–20 Hz band of its frequency spectrum, and the remainder as noise. These frequency range was considered following [12,13], where ECG

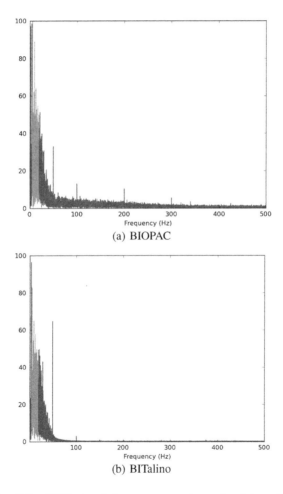

(a) BIOPAC

(b) BITalino

Fig. 3. Example of the ECG signal frequency spectrum for data collected with each acquisition device in one of the recording sessions. The blue region shows the interest spectral band and the remainder the noise (Color figure online)

was also obtained at the hands level. For each record we computed the difference between the SNR obtained from BITalino and BIOPAC acquisitions.

Figure 3 illustrates an example of the frequency spectrum of ECG data acquired in both devices, for one of the test subjects in the experiment 1. The 50 Hz power line interference is visible in both signals; however, since the BITalino ECG sensor has an analog band pass filter from 0.5 to 40 Hz, the higher frequencies are almost eliminated, contrary to what happens with the BIOPAC.

For the cosine distance calculation, the synchronized signals were segmented into individual heartbeat waveforms, and the distance between a given segment in the BIOPAC time series and the matching segment in the BITalino time series was calculated. The cosine distance, D_{cos}, between the signals x and y is given by Eq. 2

$$D_{cos}(x, y) = 1 - \frac{\sum_{k=1}^{m} x[k] y[k]}{\sqrt{\sum_{k=1}^{m} x[k]^2 \sum_{k=1}^{m} y[k]^2}}, \tag{2}$$

The reason why we have calculated the cosine distance for each heartbeat, instead of using the entire signal, is due to the fact that we were only interested in the ECG waveform shape, which is comprised in the heartbeat region. To validate the similarity between the signals acquired from the two devices, we computed the RMSE, as defined in Eq. 3

$$RMSE(x, y) = \sqrt{\frac{\sum_{j=1}^{N} \left(D_{cos_j}(x, y) \right)^2}{N}} \tag{3}$$

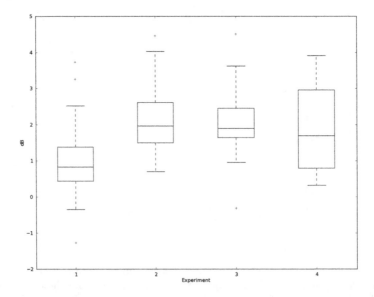

Fig. 4. Boxplot of the difference between BITalino and BIOPAC Signal-to-Noise Ratio for each experiment

5   Experimental Results

The results obtained for each experiment in the 20 subjects are represented in Fig. 4. The box plots display the distribution of the SNR differences across all subjects. The height of the box plot indicates the degree of dispersion, the band inside the box represents the median, and the bottom and top of the box are the first and third quartiles. The smallest SNR difference between devices was obtained in experiment 1, where the median value is lower and the degree of dispersion is reduced. This was already expected since the presence of the ground electrode in the BIOPAC device and the use of gelled electrodes in both systems correspond to the best case scenario in which the amount of captured noise is minimal. The higher dispersion obtained was in experiment 4, due to higher noise presence in the signals.

Table 2. Experimental results from BIOPAC and BITalino ECG signals acquisition, in the 4 experiments detailed in Table 1.

Experiment	RMSE	SNR [dB] BITalino	SNR [dB] BIOPAC
1	0.0043 ± 0.0053	-1.02 ± 2.04	-2.04 ± 2.31
2	0.0042 ± 0.0039	-1.19 ± 1.84	-3.35 ± 2.45
3	0.0063 ± 0.0055	-1.62 ± 2.21	-3.69 ± 2.54
4	0.0042 ± 0.0043	-1.87 ± 2.14	-3.80 ± 2.66

Table 2 summarizes the results obtained for the signals collected using each device. In all the experiments, the SNR of BITalino was higher than BIOPAC. This was already expected due to the analogic filtering implemented in the BITalino ECG sensor.

The lowest value of SNR with the BITalino device was obtained in experiment 4, when using the paper electrodes, indicating an higher noise presence. In what concerns the morphological correlation between waveforms, all the experiments have shown a high similarity between the ECG signals obtained from both devices. The acquired signals have a good approximation to the well known prototypical ECG waveform, providing an easy identification of the characteristic P-QRS-T complexes. Figure 5 presents an overlay with all the individual heartbeat waveforms collected in one of the recording sessions, showing the median and standard deviation of all the segments obtained from both devices in the four experiments. As we can see, the waveform morphology is maintained throughout the experiments and is virtually indistinguishable between devices and materials.

From the cosine distance results, we have calculated the RMSE, and the results are described in Table 2. For all the experiments, we verified very low RMSE values, indicating that the signals obtained from all three types of electrodes retain much of the waveform morphology when compared to the signals

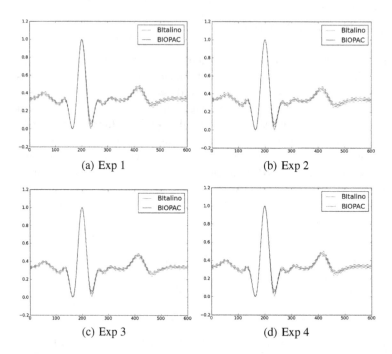

(a) Exp 1   (b) Exp 2

(c) Exp 3   (d) Exp 4

Fig. 5. Segmented heartbeat waveforms from the BITalino (blue) and the BIOPAC (grey); the solid wave represents the mean, and dashed line the standard deviation (Color figure online).

obtained with the gold standard BIOPAC setup. An interesting finding is that the inkjet printed electrodes shows a very good performance when compared to the other electrodes, with a RMSE of 0.0042, while with the dry electrodes we obtained the worst results, with a RMSE of 0.0063. Although the signals obtained with the paper-based electrodes present a lower SNR, the ECG morphology is maintained, which results in a similar performance to that found for the case in which standard clinical-grade pre-gelled Ag/AgCl electrodes are used. Moreover, the signals acquired with the BITalino device are highly correlated to those obtained with the BIOPAC, actually exhibiting lower noise levels in raw ECG signals.

6   Conclusions

In this paper we have proposed and evaluated paper-based inkjet printed electrodes for ECG data acquisition. We presented the fabrication steps, and benchmarked our electrodes against standard clinical-grade pre-gelled Ag/AgCl electrodes, and dry electrodes. Data acquisition was performed using a BIOPAC system, considered to be a gold standard within the biosignal research community, nonetheless due to the fact that it is a closed system, we have also supported our analysis on the BITalino, a physiological computing platform first introduced by our team.

Experimental results have shown that the proposed approach explored in this work achieves comparable performance in terms of SNR and RMSE when comparing with a gold standard equipment. Furthermore, our evaluation showed that the heartbeat waveforms measured through using paper-based inkjet electrodes and BITalino are nearly identical to those obtained with the BIOPAC.

We believe that our approach has a threefold advantage of reducing production costs, being easier to recycle, and being more accessible when comparing to conventional approaches. Consequently, new possibilities can be opened in the field of biosignals, enabling people (e.g. patients and/or caregivers) to have easier access to consumables in continuous ambulatory monitoring scenarios.

Acknowledgements. This work was partially funded by Fundação para a Ciência e Tecnologia (FCT) under the project grant PTDC/EEI-SII/2312/2012, and scholarships grants SFRH/BD/65248/2009 and SFRH/PROTEC/49512/2009, whose support the authors gratefully acknowledge. The authors would also thank the students form Instituto Superior Técnico and Faculdade de Ciências that were volunteers on this study.

References

1. Silva, H., Lourenço, A., Lourenço, R., Leite, P., Coutinho, D., Fred, A.: Study and evaluation of a single differential sensor design based on electro-textile electrodes for ECG biometrics applications. In: Proceedings of the IEEE Sensors Conference, pp. 1764–1767 (2011)
2. Silva, H., Carreiras, C., Lourenço, A., Fred, A.L.N.: Off-the-person electrocardiography. In: International Congress on Cardiovascular Technologies (CARDIOTECHNIX), September 2013
3. Cheng, J., Lukowicz, P., Henze, N., Schmidt, A., Amft, O., Salvatore, G., Troster, G.: Smart textiles: from niche to mainstream. IEEE Pervasive Comput. **12**(3), 81–84 (2013)
4. Marozas, V., Petrenas, A., Daukantas, S., Lukosevicius, A.: A comparison of conductive textile-based and silver/silver chloride gel electrodes in exercise electrocardiogram recordings. J. Electrocardiol. **44**(2), 189–194 (2011)
5. Chiodo, J., Ijomah, W.: Use of active disassembly technology to improve remanufacturing productivity: automotive application. Int. J. Comput. Integr. Manuf. **27**(4), 1–11 (2014)
6. Siegel, A.C., Phillips, S.T., Dickey, M.D., Lu, N., Suo, Z., Whitesides, G.M.: Foldable printed circuit boards on paper substrates. Adv. Funct. Mater. **20**(1), 28–35 (2010)
7. Leenen, M.A.M., Arning, V., Thiem, H., Steiger, J., Anselmann, R.: Printable electronics: flexibility for the future. Phys. Status Solidi A **206**(4), 588–597 (2009)
8. Tobjörk, D., Österbacka, R.: Paper electronics. Adv. Mater. **23**(17), 1935–1961 (2011)
9. Singh, M., Haverinen, H.M., Dhagat, P., Jabbour, G.E.: Inkjet printing-process and its applications. Adv. Mater. **22**(6), 673–685 (2010)

10. Calvert, P.: Inkjet printing for materials and devices. Chem. Mater. **13**(10), 3299–3305 (2001)
11. Clark, J.W., Neuman, M.R., Olson, W.H., Peura, R.A., Primiano, F.P.: Medical Instrumentation: Application and Design, 4th edn. Wiley, Hoboken (2009)
12. Alves, A.P., Silva, H., Lourenço, A., Fred, A.: BITalino: a biosignal acquisition system based on Arduino. In: Proceeding of the 6th Conference on Biomedical Electronics and Devices (BIODEVICES), pp. 261–264 (2013)
13. Guerreiro, J., Silva, H., Lourenço, A., Martins, R., Fred, A.: BITalino: a multimodal platform for physiological computing. In: Proceeding of the 10th International Conference on Informatics in Control, Automation and Robotics (ICINCO) (2013)
14. De Chazal, P., O'Dwyer, M., Reilly, R.: Automatic classification of heartbeats using ECG morphology and heartbeat interval features. IEEE Trans. Biomed. Eng. **51**(7), 1196–1206 (2004)
15. Engelse, W.A.H., Zeelenberg, C.: A single scan algorithm for QRS-detection and feature extraction. Comput. Cardiol. **6**, 37–42 (1979)

An EOG-Based Automatic Sleep Scoring System and Its Related Application in Sleep Environmental Control

Chih-En Kuo[1]([✉]), Sheng-Fu Liang[3], Yi-Chieh Lee[2], Fu-Yin Cherng[2], Wen-Chieh Lin[2], Peng-Yu Chen[3], Yen-Chen Liu[3], and Fu-Zen Shaw[1]

[1] The Institute of Cognitive Science, National Cheng Kung University, Tainan, Taiwan
chihen.kuo@gmail.com, fzshaw@mail.ncku.edu.tw
[2] Department of Computer Science, National Chiao Tung University, Tainan, Taiwan
be341341@gmail.com, fufu22710@gmail.com, wclin@cs.nctu.edu.tw
[3] Department of Computer Science and Information Engineering, National Cheng Kung University, Tainan, Taiwan
sfliang@mail.ncku.edu.tw, a13524000@gmail.com, yenchen0304@gmail.com

Abstract. Human beings spend approximately one third of their lives sleeping. Conventionally, to evaluate a subjects sleep quality, all-night polysomnogram (PSG) readings are taken and scored by a well-trained expert. Unlike a bulky PSG or EEG recorder on the head, the development of an electrooculogram (EOG)-based automatic sleep-staging system will enable physiological computing systems (PhyCS) to progress toward easy sleep and comfortable monitoring. In this paper, an EOG-based sleep scoring system is proposed. EOG signals are also coupling some of sleep characteristics of EEG signals. Compared to PSG or EEG recordings, EOG has the advantage of easy placement, and can be operated by the user individually at home. The proposed method was found to be more than 83 % accurate when compared with the manual scorings applied to sixteen subjects. In addition to sleep-quality evaluation, the proposed system encompasses adaptive brightness control of light according to online monitoring of the users sleep stages. The experiments show that the EOG-based sleep scoring system is a practicable solution for homecare and sleep monitoring due to the advantages of comfortable recording and accurate sleep staging.

Keywords: Sleep · Sleep stage · Adaptive system · Electrooculogram (EOG) · Interaction design · Sleep quality

1 Introduction

In recent years, physiologically sensing technologies have been applied to human computer interaction. They can not only help people with disabilities but also be integrated into general user interfaces used by healthy people. They also create

© Springer-Verlag Berlin Heidelberg 2014
H.P. da Silva et al. (Eds.): PhyCS 2014, LNCS 8908, pp. 71–88, 2014.
DOI: 10.1007/978-3-662-45686-6_5

more diverse interactive ways and help users keep healthy [32]. Electrooculography (EOG), which measures our eye movement, is a kind of physiological sensing technologies. Several studies in the human computer interaction (HCI) field have shown that EOG can be used to track eye gazes [4,22]. In addition to detecting eye gazes, a recent study also suggested that EOG can be used to classify people's sleep stage [36].

Sleep is important for human health. Sleep diseases, such as insomnia and obstructive sleep apnea, seriously affect quality of life. Sleep is not a static stage but a dynamic process [28]. Sleep can be divided into six periods: wakefulness (Wake); the four stages of non-rapid eye movement (NREM, numbered 1–4); and rapid eye movement (REM). Stages 3 and 4 have also been combined, and referred as the slow wave sleep stage (SWS). Conventionally, to evaluate a subjects sleep quality, all-night PSG tests including electroencephalograms (EEG), EOG, and electromyograms (EMG) are usually recorded and scored by a well-trained expert [28]. Due to their high cost and bulk, conventional PSG systems are not suitable for sleep recording at home.

The HCI field has begun to take note of sleep-related issues [1,6], and additional interaction designs to aid sleep have been proposed. Several studies identify factors that would affect sleep quality, and provide suggestions to improve it [33]. In addition to self-management, advances in interaction designs may assist users to achieve better sleep quality and habits [1]. One prior study [2] applied the concept of peripheral display to the design of mobile applications that can encourage users to keep good sleeping habits. There are also various systems using sensors on mobile phones to help users record sleep stages [19] and to understand their sleep quality. Some products focus on waking users up by adjusting light levels during the period near the preset wake-up time, e.g., the Philips Wake-up Light.

Choe et al. (2011) have indicated many factors affecting sleep quality, including caffeine, the bedroom environment, and fears. Aliakseyeu et al. (2011), meanwhile, have suggested several design opportunities for improving sleep, some of which would need the support of real-time sleep-stage monitoring. Indeed, the results of these studies inspired us to develop an automatic scoring system. Recently, several proposals have been made for phone-based applications (apps) and wearable devices to monitor sleep efficiency (wake-sleep states), using accelerometers to detect body movements during sleep. These devices are easy to use, but cannot accurately recognize sleep stages and they may not function at all if used other than in bed, e.g. while having a nap in the office. The development of an online sleep-staging system that does not require the mounting of a bulky PSG system on the head will allow PhyCS to progress toward easier sleep and more comfortable monitoring.

This paper proposes an EOG-based sleep monitoring system including EOG acquisition and a sleep-staging method based on EOG signal analysis. Compared to all-night PSG or EEG recordings, EOG has the advantage of easy placement, and can be measured by the individual user without assistance. An automatic EOG sleep-scoring method integrating the time-domain EOG feature analysis and a linear classifier is proposed. The agreement between the proposed method and the expert scoring is higher than 83 %, placing it within the range of inter-score agreement [23]. Active control of environmental light/brightness, based on online monitoring of the users sleep stages by the proposed system, is also demonstrated.

2   Background and Related Work

2.1   PhyCS for Sleep

In addition to assistive technologies for healthy living, researchers have started to develop PhyCSs that integrate sensing and computing technologies to support healthy sleep. Choe et al. (2011) conducted large-scale surveys and interviews to identify the design opportunities for supporting healthy sleep. According to their study, healthy people care almost as much about their sleep quality as insomnia patients do. Instead of clinical sleep diagnosis based on all-night PSG recording (including EEG, EOG and EMG), new portable recording devices with automatic analysis software have been developed for home applications; these include Zeo, Fitbit, and Bodymedia. In addition, a number of phone apps have been developed to help users analyze their sleep processes [19]. The main purposes of these technologies are to monitor users sleep quality and to remind them of their sleep problems. Prior study [1] has suggested some interaction designs for sleep applications, which may help people to enhance sleep quality, and accommodate the differing sleep habits of individuals.

2.2   Sleep Monitoring Devices

Recently, many novel techniques for online monitoring of physiological signals have been developed to help patients with sleep disorders [5]. Patients can wear wireless sensors that allow caregivers to monitor their conditions and provide help when needed [32]. Some products for improving sleep quality have already reached the market, and these include both sleep-management systems and sleep clocks [16]. It is reasonably clear that people have begun to pay particular attention to their sleep efficiency and quality. A sleep-management system usually consists of one or more sensors and a monitoring system (or a user interface). A user wears the sensors on their body and pre-sets up a wake-up time; the system will then wake up the user at a proper sleep stage at or before the wake-up time.

Zeo is a sleep-management product, shaped like a sports headband with three sensors attached on the forehead. Fitbit provides the user with a sleep quality score by measuring how long they sleep and how many times they wake up. Fitbit also has a silent wake-up alarm that gently vibrates to wake up the user by their preset time. The functionalities of Bodymedia Fit are similar to those of Fitbit. It lets users know the quality and efficiency of their sleep. In general, Zeo, Fitbit and Bodymedia Fit provide users with helpful information such as sleep efficiency (wake-sleep states) for sleep management; however, they may not be able to accurately recognize the whole range of sleep stages.

2.3 EOG-Based Sleep Scoring Method

Wearable EOG systems have been used for eye tracking in the past. They are easy to use and do not obscure users field of view. For example, Bulling et al. (2009) embedded an EOG system into goggles that can recognize eye gestures in real time [4]. Manaby and Fukumoto also attempted to design an all-day-wearable gaze detector based on EOG [22]. These systems show that EOG can potentially be used in our daily life.

Besides eye tracking, Virkkala et al. (2007) further proposed that EOG can be utilized to classify sleep stages effectively. The agreement between computer analysis/scoring of EOG signals, on the one hand, and the expert scoring of PSG signals is nearly 73 %. This is not in the range of inter-score agreement (>82 %, Norman et al., 2000), but if its accuracy can be improved, the EOG-based sleep staging system will be a very practicable solution for home-use sleep monitoring, due to the advantages of comfortable recording (as compared to PSG) and complete sleep staging (as compared to actigraphy).

3 An EOG-Based Automatic Sleep Scoring Method

Our EOG-based sleep-stage scoring method includes three parts: preprocessing, feature extraction, and classification. The following subsections introduce each part in greater detail.

3.1 Preprocessing

The sampling rate of our EOG signals is 256 Hz. According to Rechtschaffen and Kales (1968) (hereafter, R&K rules), the major brain activity during sleep consists of low-frequency rhythms (<30 Hz), and therefore an eighth-order Butterworth band-pass filter with a 0.5–30 Hz pass-band is used to filter the recordings for artifact rejection and enhancement of sleep-related physiological activities. Multi-scale entropy (MSE) has been used to analyze the filtered signals, as recommended by (Costa et al., 2005). In addition, an eighth-order Butterworth band-pass filter with a 4–8 Hz pass-band is utilized to extract the theta band components for the autoregressive (AR) model, as recommended by [26].

3.2 Feature Extraction

Our feature extraction process includes: (a) MSE, (b) AR modeling, and (c) multi-scale line length (MLL). The MSE is the principal foundation of the method; the AR model and the MLL are complementary features for increasing the classification accuracy of S1 and REM.

(a) **Multi-scale Entropy.** MSE is a signal-analysis method recently proposed by Costa et al. (2005). It estimates the complexity associated with the long-range temporal correlation of a time series. Instead of using a single scale, MSE measures the complexity of a time series by considering entropy at multiple temporal scales. MSE has been used to analyze the complexity of various biomedical signals such as EEG [15,20,34], ECG [7], and heart rate [8,24].

Given an EOG time series with N samples, $x = \{x_1, x_2, x_3, \cdots, x_N\}$, the original time series is divided into non-overlapping time windows of length τ, which is defined as the scale factor. A coarse-gained time series $y_\tau(j)$ is then calculated by averaging the data points inside a time window,

$$y_\tau(j) = \frac{1}{\tau} \sum_{i=(j-1)\tau+1}^{j\tau} x_i, \ 1 \le j \le \left\lfloor \frac{N}{\tau} \right\rfloor \tag{1}$$

After obtaining each element of the coarse-gained time series for each scale τ, the entropy of each coarse-gained time series is calculated. Theoretically, if the complexity of the signal is greater, the entropy value will be higher. Relatively, the entropy value is smaller. Two popular approaches for physiological time series analysis are approximate entropy (ApEn) [27] and sample entropy (SampEn) [29]. SampEn was proposed to overcome some limitations of ApEn, such as bias caused by incorrect counting of self-matches to avoid the occurrence of a natural logarithm of zero in the calculation. Therefore, in this paper, SampEn has been utilized to calculate the entropy of the EOG time series. More details of SampEn can be found in Richman and Moorman (2000). The windows of length τ are set as 1–8, and therefore we have eight entropy values corresponding to different time resolutions, extracted as the features after MSE analysis.

(b) Autoregressive Model. An AR model is a parametric model used to describe a stationary time series. It is a popular tool for EEG analysis [3,25,35]. AR models represent the current value of a time series $x(t)$ as the weighted sum of its previous values $x(t - i)$ and an uncorrelated error $\varepsilon(t)$,

$$x(t) = \sum_{i=1}^{p} a_i x(t - i) + \varepsilon(t), \tag{2}$$

where $a(i)$ is the AR coefficients and p is the order of the AR model. In this paper, we compute $a(i)$ and p from the theta band signals (4–8 Hz) extracted by an eighth-order Butterworth band-pass filter in the preprocessing phase. The computed $a(i)$ and p are used to determine EOG states.

(c) Multi-scale line length. MLL calculates the line length for each coarse-gained time series. The line length LL of a time series is the sum of the vertical distance (absolute difference) between successive samples of the time series [9],

$$LL = \frac{1}{N-1} \sum_{i=1}^{N-1} |x_{i+1} - x_i|, \tag{3}$$

where x is the time series considered, i represents the temporal index of the time series, and N is the total length of the time series.

Line length reflects changes of waveform dimensionality and is a measurement sensitive to variations of signal amplitude and frequency [13]. MLL has the advantage of low computational complexity and is therefore suitable for online applications. It has also been used for automatic epileptic-seizure detection in EEG [9].

A total of 24 features, including 13 MSE values, eight AR coefficients, and three MLL values are extracted from the EOG signals and fed in to a linear classifier for sleep-stage classification.

3.3   Classifier

Due to its low computational cost, we chose to utilize linear discriminant analysis (LDA) to classify five sleep stages based on the extracted MSE values, AR coefficients and MLL values. In addition, we wanted to ensure that the proposed EOG features were effective to a point that sleep stages could be determined simply using a linear classifier.

(a) **Linear discriminant analysis.** LDA finds a hyperplane that best separates two or more classes of objects or events by adjusting the linear weighting of their features. Usually, the within-class, between-class, and mixture scatter matrices are used to formulate the criteria for searching the hyperplane [17,21]. In order to test the generalization ability of the proposed method, the EOG data of 16 subjects were used to train the LDA classifier, while the EOG data of a different group of 16 subjects were used to verify the performance of our proposed method.

(b) **Smoothing.** Sleep-stage scoring has periodicity and continuity from light to deep (R&K rules). After classifying the sleep stage using LDA, some misclassified epochs can be corrected according to temporal contextual information and R&K rules, which refer to the relation between epochs prior and posterior to the current epoch. For example, three consecutive epochs consisting of S2, REM, and S2 should be followed by the sequence S2, S2, S2. Similarly, consecutive epochs of REM, S1 and REM should be followed by the sequence REM, REM, REM. Following the protocols established by Iber (2007) and Virkkala et al. (2007) [14,36], a total of 10 rules were utilized to smooth the final results and increase the accuracy of our method.

4   Sleep-Stage Scoring Experiment

4.1   Subjects and Recordings

All-night PSG sleep recordings were obtained from 32 healthy subjects (18 males and 14 females) ranging in age from 18 to 24 years. The subjects were interviewed about their sleep quality and medical history. Their sleep efficiency ranged from 56 % to 97 %. None of them reported any history of neurological or psychological disorders. The PSG recordings of each subject were made using six EEG channels (F3-A2, F4-A1, C3-A2, C4-A1, P3-A2, and P4-A1, following the international 10–20 standard system), two EOG channels (the above-right and below-left outer canthus), and a chin EMG channel, and were acquired through the Siesta 802

PSG (Compumedics, Inc.). The sampling rate was 256 Hz with 16-bit resolution. The filter settings of the cut-off frequencies were 0.5–30 Hz for EEG/EOG, and 5–100 Hz for EMG. These nine-channel signals were used for manual scoring, as suggested by the R&K rules, whereas only the EOG data were used for the single-channel sleep-stage scoring system being developed.

The 32 PSG sleep recordings were visually scored by a sleep specialist using the R&K rules. Each 30-s epoch was classified into Wake, REM, S1, S2, SWS, and movement artifacts. In our experiments, only epochs of the five sleep stages were used; epochs of movement artifacts were rejected [3,31].

4.2 Performance Evaluation

Next, we evaluated the performance of our automatic EOG-based sleep-scoring method. The performance criterion was the agreement between computer scoring, on the one hand, and expert scoring based on all PSG channels. The proposed systems sensitivity corresponding to each sleep stage is shown in Table 1. The rows represent the results arrived at by the experts visual scoring, and the columns represent the results of our method. The sensitivities of the proposed automatic stage-scoring method that were associated with the five sleep stages were 81.45 % (Wake), 28.05 % (S1), 88.12 % (S2), 83.06 % (SWS) and 81.05 % (REM), yielding an overall sensitivity of 83.33 %. The sensitivities for all stages except for S1 were higher than 81 %. S1 can easily be mis-categorized as any of the other stages except SWS, and the number of S1 epochs is significantly lower than that of other stages epochs. As such, it is difficult to create a model with a high sensitivity for S1. Rosenberg et al. [30] report that inter-scorer agreement in a large group is approximately 83 % under current manual scoring rules, a level similar to that reported for agreement between expert scorers.

Comparing the recognition results achieved by the present study against the existing, purely EOG-based sleep-stage scoring method proposed by [36], overall agreement has increased from 73 % to 83 %. The results of the method in Virkkala et al. are Wake, 79.7 %; S1, 30.6 %; S2, 79.7 %; SWS, 75.9 %; and REM, 75.6 %. As detailed in the preceding paragraph, our method performed better in four of the five stages (Wake, S2, SWS, and REM), and with regard to the remaining stage, the results are similar (28 % vs. 30.6 %).

5 Lighting Control System Based on Sleep Stages

In addition to sleep quality evaluation, it is worth considering whether a comfortable sleep monitor can be utilized to control the sleep environment. Accordingly, the present research also incorporated an active brightness-control system governed by online monitoring of the users sleep stages.

People can now purchase various lighting products that mimic the effect of natural sunlight. For example, the Philips Wake-up Light© is a dawn-simulation product that allows users to set up their wake-up time, the period of dawn or dusk simulation, and the maximal light intensity. This and other dawn-dusk

Table 1. Confusion matrix of five-stage classification comparing the proposed EOG-based sleep scoring and manual sleep scoring based on PSG recordings.

	EOG system	Wake	S1	S2	SWS	REM	SE(%)
Expert	Wake	1094	55	33	11	150	81.45
	S1	100	124	76	8	134	28.05
	S2	28	203	5880	380	177	88.18
	SWS	5	1	376	1884	2	83.06
	REM	39	326	116	2	2129	81.05
	Overall						83.33
	Kappa						0.75

simulation products gradually modify light intensity to simulate natural ambient light and help users fall sleep and/or wake up [10–12]. However, these dawn-dusk simulation products do not take any account of the users sleep stages. In particular, since every persons sleep pattern is different and may vary from time to time, changing light intensity according to a preset fixed program may not be appropriate, and even disturb a users sleeping partners who have different bedtime or wake-up time. Hence, it is desirable to develop an adaptive system that can dynamically adjust its lighting to let each user sleep and wake up gradually and individually.

5.1 System Requirements and Design Concept

In order to extend the PhyCSs-based sleep analysis for actively controlling the sleep environment, we have developed a lighting-control system that adaptively varies its brightness based on the users sleep stage. Following on from the discussion in the previous section, our system was intended fulfill the following requirements: (a) Use online technology to classify a users sleep stages; (b) Use online technology to adjust the lighting of the sleep environment according to the users sleep stages; (c) During hours of darkness, provide faint light when the user wakes up and moves, to avoid falling; (d) Wake up the user during a proper sleep stage (i.e. S1, S2 and REM) at or before the user-specified wake-up time; and (e) Record and provide sleep information including sleep period, total sleep time, sleep latency, and sleep efficiency so that the user can learn about their sleep pattern. Figure 1 shows the concept and architecture of our adaptive light system. The processing steps were as follows:

1. A portable wireless EOG recording unit was used to record the users sleep EOG online.
2. The EOG signal was sent to a personal computer via wireless transmission.
3. An automatic sleep-scoring method based on EOG signals was utilized to classify the users sleep stage online. The output of the automatic sleep-scoring method is the users current sleep stage.

4. According to the users current sleep stage, the lighting-control algorithm gradually adjusts the brightness of light. The lighting-control algorithm also considers the situation of the user moving about during the night, e.g. to go to the toilet, and supplies adequate lighting to avoid falls.

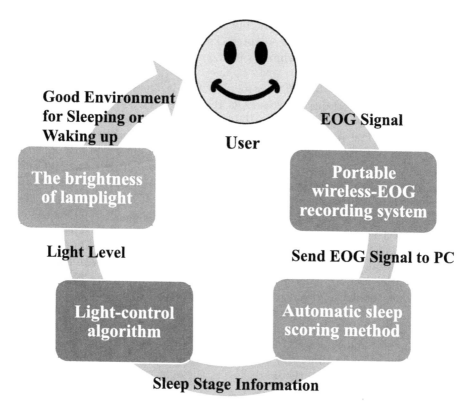

Fig. 1. The concept and architecture of the proposed adaptive light system.

5.2   Portable Wireless EOG Recording Unit

In our design concept, a portable wireless EOG recording unit (as shown in Fig. 2) is integrated with our sleep-scoring system to perform online sleep-stage monitoring. It consists of three components: Part A is a CC2530 wireless sender; Part B is the amplifier circuit of electrocardiography; and Part C is a CC2530 wireless adapter. Because the device is designed for online automatic sleep-stage scoring, most of the signals are in the low frequency band. Therefore, we chose the range of 0.3–35 Hz as the passband of the analog filter. This system can continuously operate for, at most, 30 h.

5.3 Control Module

Our lighting-control module consists of a circuit board with micro-controller and a sleep-stage-based lighting-control algorithm to control the brightness of an LED bulb. The circuit board we used is *Arduino Uno*, which has a micro-controller with a 16 MHz clock rate and 14 digital I/O pins (of which six provide PWM output). It can be connected to a computer via a USB cable for both data transmission and power supply, but it can also be run on a stand-alone basis, powered via an AC-to-DC adapter. The specifications of the LED bulb are, Color temperature: warm white 3500 K; current: 700 mA; voltage: 3.2–3.7 v; brightness: 130–150 lm.

Our sleep-stage-based lighting control algorithm is illustrated in Fig. 3. When the user wears our portable wireless-EOG recording unit and goes to bed, the brightness decreases from 200 lux to 100 lux over the course of 90 s. When the users sleep stage first reaches S1, the brightness decreases from 100 lux to 50 lux over a period of 150 s. Similarly, when users sleep stage enters its first S2, the brightness decreases from 50 lux to 25 lux in 60 s. The light is turned off 60 s after users sleep stage enters its first SWS epoch. Then, if the user appears to experience three continuous Wake epochs, indicating that they are likely to get up, the algorithm turns on the light and the brightness increases to 50 lux in 5 s. When the user goes to sleep again, the lighting control algorithm would check the first S2 and SWS, and the light is turned off gradually again. On the other hand, if the users sleep stage does not show three consecutive Wake epochs, it means that the user has continued sleeping. Five minutes before the user-set wake-up time, the lighting control algorithm checks the users sleep stage. If the users stage is Wake, the brightness increases to 255 lux in 60 s. If, on the other hand, the users stage is S1, S2, or REM, the brightness increases to 255 lux in 300 s. If there are no Wake, S2, or REM stages within the 10 min immediately preceding the wake-up time, the brightness also increases to 255 lux in 300 s. The voice alarm rings when the brightness of the light reaches 255 lux.

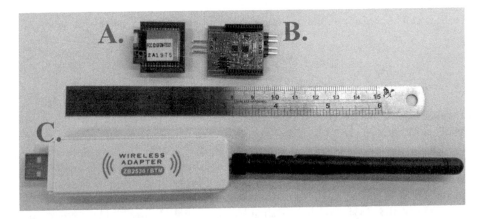

Fig. 2. The three components of the portable wireless-EOG recording unit.

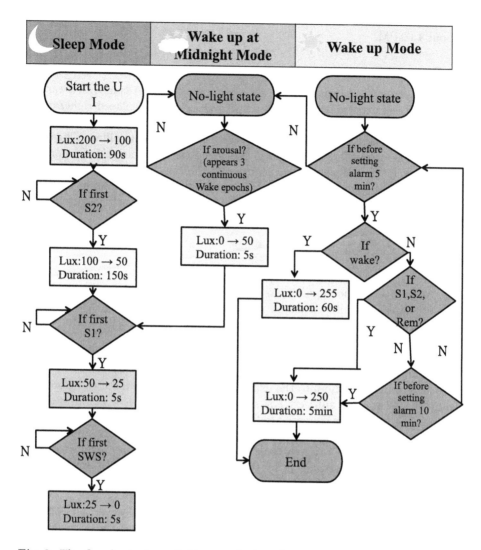

Fig. 3. The flowchart of our light control algorithm, which has three modes: sleep, wake up at the middle of the night, and wake up.

6   Lighting Control Experiment

We recruited three male subjects aged 23 ± 1.1 years old via the Internet. All three subjects had a habit of taking a nap at noon. They were asked about their sleep quality. None of them reported any history of sleep disorders. They were instructed to keep a regular sleep-wake schedule for three days prior to the experiment. Subjects were required to abstain from caffeine and alcohol throughout the course of the study. All subjects gave written informed consent before entering the study and were paid for their participation. The experiment began at about 1:00 PM.

6.1 Procedure

A darkened, quiet room was built for the sleep experiment. A camcorder was set up to record the experimental process. Two EOG channels, placed right/above and left/below outer canthus, were connected to our portable wireless EOG recording unit. The LED blub was placed next to the subjects pillow. The total sleep time was 80 min for each subject, this being the usual length of a persons first sleep cycle. Usually, sleep stages are not stable in the first sleep cycle; in particular, they change more frequently in the first sleep cycle than in the later cycles. Therefore, our experimental design focused on the first sleep cycle to verify the stability of the system in more difficult cases.

6.2 Results

In Fig. 4, (a)–(c) show the sleep hypnograms and light levels for subjects 1, 2, and 3, respectively. The experiments of all subjects can be deemed successful, as the light was gradually turned off when their sleep stage changed from Wake to SWS, and was turned on when they woke up or were in the light sleep stage 10 min before the pre-set wake-up time.

From Fig. 4(a), one can observe that brightness decreased at the beginning of sleep and during the first S1, S2, and SWS stages. The brightness of light remained zero until 71 min into the experiment, that is, nine minutes before the wake-up time set by the subject. The sleep stage of Subject 1 at 71 min was S2. Therefore, the brightness increased to 255 lux over the following 5 min. However, some Wake stages did appear between 30 min and 70 min, but all were less than three epochs in length. They may have been caused by body movement without awareness, or by misclassification by the sleep-scoring method. In any case, as these periods were less than three consecutive epochs, the light did not turn on. The results from Subject 2 were similar to those of Subject 1.

Figure 4(c) shows that Subject 3 achieved SWS quickly; however, he woke up two times between the 39-min mark and the 51-min mark. Our system provided faint light for purposes of safety when the user woke up, and turned off again when his sleep stage had returned to SWS. It is worth mentioning that the sleep stage of Subject 3 changed quickly between minute 40 and minute 60. Such rapid changes of sleep stage often result in incorrect sleep-stage scoring. To avoid mistakenly turning on the light when it is not needed, the lighting control algorithm may be adjusted according to a users sleep pattern and efficiency. Other factors affecting the sleep environment, such as music and temperature, can also be considered in the future.

7 Discussion

Comfortable recording and accurate sleep-stage classification are two essential criteria for sensing and computing technologies designed to support healthy sleep.

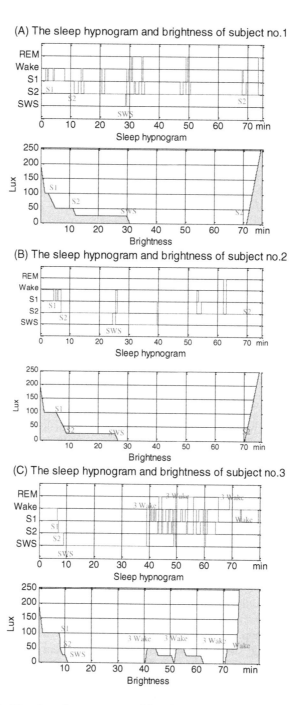

Fig. 4. The sleep hypnogram and brightness of the three subjects.

Due to their high cost and bulk, conventional PSG systems are not suitable for sleep recording at home. Expert scoring of PSG recordings is also a time-consuming process. Recently developed phone apps and wearable devices for sleep monitoring are easy to use, but none claim to accurately recognize the full range of sleep stages. In this paper, an EOG-based sleep-scoring system has been proposed. Compared to PSG or EEG recordings, our EOG-based device has the advantage of easy placement and can be operated by the individual user with minimal training. The accuracy of the proposed method as compared with manual scoring can reach 83.33 %. This solution balances the criteria of comfortable recording and accurate sleep staging.

In addition to sleep-quality evaluation, our system incorporates active light control. Our results demonstrate that light can be adjusted automatically based on the sleep stages of human subjects. Sleep hypnograms show that the time-points of different subjects sleep stages from awake to light sleep or from light sleep to deep sleep were very different. Hence, a dawn-dusk simulation should ideally control the brightness of light based on the users sleep stage, in order to overcome individual differences in their sleep patterns.

Prior work [6] indicated that users were not accustomed to wearing biosensors while asleep. This suggests that we must improve the comfort of this type of device in the future. Furthermore, there is lack of long-term (i.e. month-long or longer) studies of the use of portable sleep-monitoring devices in daily life [10]. With improvements to devices and increased user familiarity, negative user experiences can be expected to decrease.

7.1   Benefits of Adaptive System

Most of the existing work in this area [16,19] only recorded users sleep stages and helped them to analyze their sleep quality, without providing an active system to modulate the sleeping environment appropriately in harmony with users individual sleep stages.

Kupfer and Reynolds (1997) indicated that television was seen as a cause of disrupted sleep [18]. However, it may help those who fear sleeping alone, or who need to be shielded from outside noise [1,6]. An adaptive system similar to the one we propose could adjust the brightness and contrast of TV screens to guide users to sleep, and shut down the TV automatically when users fall asleep. Since it has been demonstrated that lights can be adjusted and turned on and off automatically based on individuals sleep stages in real time, adaptive lighting adjustment could also help children who are afraid of the dark. A sleeping environment that is actively attuned to users sleep stages will allow them to have a better quality of sleep.

Besides improving sleep quality, an adaptive system might bring other benefits. For example, users could show their sleep stages to flight attendants on long air journeys, so that the flight attendants could avoid disrupting their rest when they are in deep sleep. For users who sleep with a partner, timely detection of sleep stages could modulate the sleeping environment appropriately, for example by adjusting the light level and TV volume once the partner is asleep.

These automatic control systems need further design work and verification, but are certainly worthy of future research exploration.

7.2 Limitations

Our system still has some limitations. First, new EOG recording devices that can be easily worn would have to be developed if extensive use of our system was to be made. A long-term sleep monitoring system should be evaluated in the near future. Second, there is still much scope for improvement of the lighting-control algorithm, which can and should be fine-tuned to suit different subjects and scenarios. The last but not the least, our system only can monitor one people. The sleep pattern of everyone is so differ that it is very difficult to control the sleep environment to meet everyone. Actually, the people with some sleep problems was recommend to sleep alone for avoiding the noise from other people.

8   Conclusions

This paper proposed a comfortable, accurate EOG-based sleep-monitoring system. In addition to off-line sleep quality evaluation, its usefulness extends to dynamic control of light levels based on users sleep stages. This study demonstrates the feasibility of using online and closed-loop PhyCS to control a sleeping environment adaptively.

It is hoped that this work may open up new research horizons and strategies with regard to both sleep monitoring and environmental control. When a comfortable online sleep monitor is available, this system can be utilized to control the sleep environment for easy sleep. A system that automatically and adaptively adjusts environmental factors based on a users sleep stages for the purpose of sleep quality enhancement is feasible.

Acknowledgements. This work was supported by the National Science Council of Taiwan under Grants NSC 102-2221-E-009-082-MY3, 100-2410-H-006-025-MY3, and 1102-2220-E-006-001. Moreover, this paper was also supported by "Aiming for the Top University Program" of the National Chiao Tung University and Ministry of Education,Taiwan, R.O.C.

References

1. Aliakseyeu, D., Du, J., Zwartkruis-Pelgrim, E., Subramanian, S.: Exploring interaction strategies in the context of sleep. In: Campos, P., Graham, N., Jorge, J., Nunes, N., Palanque, P., Winckler, M. (eds.) INTERACT 2011, Part III. LNCS, vol. 6948, pp. 19–36. Springer, Heidelberg (2011)
2. Bauer, J., Consolvo, S., Greenstein, B., Schooler, J., Wu, E., Watson, N.F., Kientz, J., Bauer, J.S.: Shuteye: encouraging awareness of healthy sleep recommendations with a mobile, peripheral display. In: Proceedings of the 2012 ACM Annual Conference on Human Factors in Computing Systems, pp. 1401–1410. ACM (2012)

3. Berthomier, C., Drouot, X., Herman-Stoïca, M., Berthomier, P., Prado, J., Bokar-Thire, D., Benoit, O., Mattout, J., d'Ortho, M.P.: Automatic analysis of single-channel sleep eeg: validation in healthy individuals. Sleep **30**(11), 1587 (2007)

4. Bulling, A., Roggen, D., Tröster, G.: Wearable EOG goggles: eye-based interaction in everyday environments. ACM (2009)

5. Chandra, H., Oakley, I., Silva, H.: Designing to support prescribed home exercises: understanding the needs of physiotherapy patients. In: Proceedings of the 7th Nordic Conference on Human-Computer Interaction: Making Sense Through Design, pp. 607–616. ACM (2012)

6. Choe, E.K., Consolvo, S., Watson, N.F., Kientz, J.A.: Opportunities for computing technologies to support healthy sleep behaviors. In: Proceedings of the SIGCHI Conference on Human Factors in Computing Systems, pp. 3053–3062. ACM (2011)

7. Costa, M., Goldberger, A.L., Peng, C.K.: Multiscale entropy analysis of biological signals. Phys. Rev. E **71**(2), 021906 (2005)

8. Costa, M., Peng, C.K., Goldberger, A.L., Hausdorff, J.M.: Multiscale entropy analysis of human gait dynamics. Physica A Stat. Mech. Appl. **330**(1), 53–60 (2003)

9. Esteller, R., Echauz, J., Tcheng, T., Litt, B., Pless, B.: Line length: an efficient feature for seizure onset detection. In: Proceedings of the 23rd Annual International Conference of the IEEE Engineering in Medicine and Biology Society, 2001, vol. 2, pp. 1707–1710. IEEE (2001)

10. Gasio, F.P., Kräuchi, K., Cajochen, C., van Someren, E., Amrhein, I., Pache, M., Savaskan, E., Wirz-Justice, A.: Dawn-dusk simulation light therapy of disturbed circadian rest-activity cycles in demented elderly. Exp. Gerontol. **38**(1), 207–216 (2003)

11. Fromm, E., Horlebein, C., Meergans, A., Niesner, M., Randler, C.: Evaluation of a dawn simulator in children and adolescents. Biol. Rhythm Res. **42**(5), 417–425 (2011)

12. Giménez, M.C., Hessels, M., van de Werken, M., de Vries, B., Beersma, D.G., Gordijn, M.C.: Effects of artificial dawn on subjective ratings of sleep inertia and dim light melatonin onset. Chronobiol. Int. **27**(6), 1219–1241 (2010)

13. Guo, L., Rivero, D., Dorado, J., Rabunal, J.R., Pazos, A.: Automatic epileptic seizure detection in eegs based on line length feature and artificial neural networks. J. Neurosci. Methods **191**(1), 101–109 (2010)

14. Iber, C.: The aasm manual for the scoring of sleep and associated events: rules, terminology and technical specifications (2007)

15. Kang, X., Jia, X., Geocadin, R.G., Thakor, N.V., Maybhate, A.: Multiscale entropy analysis of eeg for assessment of post-cardiac arrest neurological recovery under hypothermia in rats. IEEE Trans. Biomed. Eng. **56**(4), 1023–1031 (2009)

16. Kay, M., Choe, E.K., Shepherd, J., Greenstein, B., Watson, N., Consolvo, S., Kientz, J.A.: Lullaby: a capture & access system for understanding the sleep environment. In: Proceedings of the 2012 ACM Conference on Ubiquitous Computing, pp. 226–234. ACM (2012)

17. Kuo, B.C., Landgrebe, D.A.: Nonparametric weighted feature extraction for classification. IEEE Trans. Geosci. Remote Sens. **42**(5), 1096–1105 (2004)

18. Kupfer, D.J., Reynolds, C.F.: Management of insomnia. N. Engl. J. Med. **336**(5), 341–346 (1997)

19. Lawson, S., Jamison-Powell, S., Garbett, A., Linehan, C., Kucharczyk, E., Verbaan, S., Rowland, D.A., Morgan, K.: Validating a mobile phone application for the everyday, unobtrusive, objective measurement of sleep. In: Proceedings of the SIGCHI Conference on Human Factors in Computing Systems, pp. 2497–2506. ACM (2013)

20. Liang, S.F., Kuo, C.E., Hu, Y.H., Pan, Y.H., Wang, Y.H.: Automatic stage scoring of single-channel sleep eeg by using multiscale entropy and autoregressive models. IEEE Trans. Instrum. Meas. **61**(6), 1649–1657 (2012)

21. Lin, C.T., Ken-Li, L., Li-Wei, K., Sheng-Fu, L., Bor-Chen, K., et al.: Nonparametric single-trial eeg feature extraction and classification of driver's cognitive responses. EURASIP J. Adv. Signal Process. **2008**, 1–11 (2008)

22. Manabe, H., Fukumoto, M.: Full-time wearable headphone-type gaze detector. In: CHI'06 Extended Abstracts on Human Factors in Computing Systems, pp. 1073–1078. ACM (2006)

23. Norman, R.G., Pal, I., Stewart, C., Walsleben, J.A., Rapoport, D.M.: Interobserver agreement among sleep scorers from different centers in a large dataset. Sleep **23**(7), 901–908 (2000)

24. Norris, P.R., Anderson, S.M., Jenkins, J.M., Williams, A.E., Morris Jr., J.A.: Heart rate multiscale entropy at three hours predicts hospital mortality in 3,154 trauma patients. Shock **30**(1), 17–22 (2008)

25. Olbrich, E., Achermann, P., Meier, P.: Dynamics of human sleep eeg. Neurocomputing **52**, 857–862 (2003)

26. Pardey, J., Roberts, S., Tarassenko, L.: A review of parametric modelling techniques for eeg analysis. Med. Eng. Phys. **18**(1), 2–11 (1996)

27. Pincus, S.: Approximate entropy (apen) as a complexity measure. Chaos Interdisc. J. Nonlinear Sci. **5**(1), 110–117 (1995)

28. Rechtschaffen, A., Kales, A.: A manual of standardized terminology, techniques and scoring system for sleep stages of human subjects (1968)

29. Richman, J.S., Moorman, J.R.: Physiological time-series analysis using approximate entropy and sample entropy. Am. J. Physiol. Heart Circulatory Physiol. **278**(6), H2039–H2049 (2000)

30. Rosenberg, R.S., Van Hout, S., et al.: The american academy of sleep medicine inter-scorer reliability program: sleep stage scoring. J. Clin. Sleep Med. **9**(1), 81–87 (2013). JCSM: Official Publication of the American Academy of Sleep Medicine

31. Schaltenbrand, N., Lengelle, R., Toussaint, M., Luthringer, R., Carelli, G., Jacqmin, A., Lainey, E., Muzet, A., Macher, J.P., et al.: Sleep stage scoring using the neural network model: comparison between visual and automatic analysis in normal subjects and patients. Sleep **19**(1), 26 (1996)

32. Silva, H., Palma, S., Gamboa, H.: Aal+: Continuous institutional and home care through wireless biosignal monitoring systems. In: Bos, L., Dumay, A., Goldschmidt, L., Verhenneman, G., Yogesan, K. (eds.) Handbook of Digital Homecare, pp. 115–142. Springer, Heidelberg (2011)

33. Stepanski, E.J., Wyatt, J.K.: Use of sleep hygiene in the treatment of insomnia. Sleep Med. Rev. **7**(3), 215–225 (2003)

34. Takahashi, T., Cho, R.Y., Murata, T., Mizuno, T., Kikuchi, M., Mizukami, K., Kosaka, H., Takahashi, K., Wada, Y.: Age-related variation in eeg complexity to photic stimulation: a multiscale entropy analysis. Clin. Neurophysiol. **120**(3), 476–483 (2009)

35. Thakor, N.V., Tong, S.: Advances in quantitative electroencephalogram analysis methods. Annu. Rev. Biomed. Eng. **6**, 453–495 (2004)
36. Virkkala, J., Hasan, J., Värri, A., Himanen, S.L., Müller, K.: Automatic sleep stage classification using two-channel electrooculography. J. Neurosci. Methods **166**(1), 109–115 (2007)

Applications

Upper Body Joint Angle Measurements for Physical Rehabilitation Using Visual Feedback

Marília Barandas[1](✉), Hugo Gamboa[1], and José Manuel Fonseca[2]

[1] Physics Department, FCT-UNL, 2829-516 Caparica, Portugal
m.barandas@campus.fct.unl.pt, h.gamboa@fct.unl.pt
[2] Department of Electrotechnical Engineering,
FCT-UNL, 2829-516 Caparica, Portugal
jmrf@fct.unl.pt

Abstract. In clinical rehabilitation, biofeedback increases patient's motivation making it one of the most effective motor rehabilitation mechanisms. In this field, it is very helpful for the patient and even for the therapist to know the level of success and performance of the training process. New rehabilitation technologies allow new forms of therapy for patients with Range of Motion (ROM) disorders. The aim of this work is to introduce a simple biofeedback system in a clinical environment for ROM measurements, since there is currently a lack of practical and cost-efficient methods available for this purpose. The Microsoft Kinect™ introduces the possibility of low cost, non intrusive human motion analysis in the rehabilitation field. In this paper we conduct a comparison study of the accuracy in the computation of ROM measurements between the Kinect™ Skeleton Tracking provided by Microsoft and the proposed algorithm based on depth analysis. Experimental results showed that our algorithm is able to overcome the limitations of the Microsoft algorithm when the pose estimation is used as a measuring system making it a valuable rehabilitation tool.

Keywords: Biofeedback · Depth camera · Range of motion

1 Introduction

Biofeedback is one of the most effective motor rehabilitation mechanisms by involving the user in the evaluation of his progress and increasing his motivation [1]. In motor rehabilitation it is very important for both the patient and the therapist, to know the level of success and performance of the training process. Feedback can be divided into two categories: intrinsic and extrinsic feedback. Intrinsic feedback is generated by the movement itself, proprioception or vision of the moving limb. On the other hand, extrinsic or augmented feedback may be provided by an outside source, such as a therapist [1]. We are interested on improving the extrinsic biofeedback, since it is important for learning some

© Springer-Verlag Berlin Heidelberg 2014
H.P. da Silva et al. (Eds.): PhyCS 2014, LNCS 8908, pp. 91–104, 2014.
DOI: 10.1007/978-3-662-45686-6_6

motor tasks. Furthermore, when patients know about their progress, usually this is translated into an increase of their motivation. Some researchers claim that a growth in motivation is translated into a greater effort during task practice [1]. Pursuing and achieving goals are good reasons to keep patients motivated. Therefore, the required measurements to compare the current status with the desired goals are easily achieved by a biofeedback equipment.

Several equipments for the study of the human movement can be found on the market. However, these equipments present significant limitations when used in rehabilitation processes involving biofeedback. The most common technologies used for the human movement analysis are optical, magnetic and inertial systems. Despite that these systems usually have high accuracy and sensitivity, they also present limitations related with the complexity, space requirements, cumbersome cables carried by the patient or limited accuracy due to magnetic field distortions [2,3]. Depth cameras have been developed for several years with limitations such as low resolution, low sensitivity resulting in high noise levels and significant background noise. Until 2010, year that Microsoft and PrimeSense released the Kinect^{TM} sensor, laser scans and structured light approaches were not able to provide high frame rates for full images with a reasonable resolution. Contrary to other depth cameras, Microsoft Kinect^{TM} has low price, making it a very desirable system. Moreover, as we will see, Kinect^{TM} has good technical characteristics providing reliable depth measurements under a large variety of conditions [4]. Therefore, Microsoft Kinect^{TM}, that is used in this work, is able to overcome the limitations of existing systems and recently gained the attention of several researches due to its low cost, portability and markless anatomical measurements.

As musculoskeletal disorders are one of the most frequent injuries treated by physiotherapists and patients with these disorders usually have problems related with ROM, the introduction of a rehabilitation system based on an easy to install and operate equipment can represent a breakthrough in this clinical area.

2   Related Work

Due to the potential of the Kinect^{TM} sensor, its applications have been quite diverse. However, before using the Kinect^{TM} sensor for real applications, its 3D depth accuracy should be evaluated. Tilak Dutta [3] and Kourosh Khoshelham et al. [5] studied the 3D depth accuracy obtaining results in agreement with Microsoft's advertising. These studies also showed that Kinect^{TM} provides a depth accuracy from a few millimetres at short distance up to about 4 cm at the maximum range of the sensor.

For clinical applications, the studies made with the Kinect^{TM} sensor typically take advantage of the specific software developed by PrimeSense or Microsoft [6–9]. These systems are able to provide joint positions in real-time of 15 or 20 anatomical landmarks depending on the software used. The Kinect^{TM} sensor is usually compared with benchmark references showing that the Kinect^{TM} provides comparable data to the reference system but only in a controlled body posture.

Moreover, limitations related with the scenario are also identified. Depending on the background characteristics, sometimes the depth based skeleton reconstruction recognizes background objects as part of the subject's body.

We believe that the algorithms developed by Microsoft and PrimeSense for skeleton tracking are useful for some applications. However, when the required pose occludes some body parts or when the precision of the ROM measurements is required, these algorithms are insufficient. As this software is proprietary and closed source, it is not possible to adapt it to our needs nor extend it or improve its abilities. To overcome these problems some researchers are working with the depth information to create their own modules. In [10] the authors created their own tracking module using the depth sensing data obtained from the Kinect^{TM}. However they only detected and tracked the head, the shoulders and the hands, which is insufficient to do ROM measurements. Thus, we propose to measure them working directly with the depth map information to get a better approximation of the joints positions.

3   Instrumentation

In the following points there is a description of the sensors used during this research. The reference system chosen to validate the data from the Kinect^{TM} sensor was a triaxial accelerometer.

3.1   MotionPlux

The triaxial accelerometer used in this work was the MotionPlux [11]. This sensor, that was used as an inclinometer, is able to measure the inclination of a body segment in relation to the vertical line. This system is portable, small sized and has a sampling frequency of 800 Hz. It can be attached to a body segment without interposing with the subject's movements. A triaxial accelerometer measures the total acceleration acting in the body segment, inclination and direction of the inclination [12]. The real-time data acquired is transmitted via bluetooth to a computer and then analysed.

3.2   Kinect^{TM} Sensor

The Kinect^{TM} depth sensor has a good working range (800 to 4000 millimetres range) combined with a 16 bits pixel depth resolution, a reasonable spatial resolution (640 × 480 pixel images) and a maximum frame rate of 30 Hz. It combines this depth sensor with a 640 × 480 RGB camera sharing the field of view that is 57° on the horizontal and 43° on the vertical. Therefore, it is possible to combine the information obtained from the depth image, like joint positions and angles, with the colour images providing real-time feedback about the movements performed. The technique behind the Kinect^{TM} is based on structured-light 3D scanning and is described as a triangulation process by its inventors [5].

4   Methods

In this section, technical aspects of the capture sessions and the studied movements are presented. The method used to process the data from the Kinetic and from the reference system, as well as the comparison between them, are also shown.

4.1   Procedures

In the tests executed to validate the algorithms, the Kinect^{TM} sensor was positioned in front of the subjects at an approximate distance of 2 m. Behind the subjects there was a static flat wall. Although the wall is the best environment to do the acquisitions, one may also use other kinds of environments as long as their surfaces are not dark, shiny and rough. The MotionPlux system was attached to the subject's arm aligned with the humerus with the positive Y axis pointing the roof.

In this work, we have concentrated our study on the upper body movements belonging to common physical therapies. These movements were abduction, flexion, extension and internal and external rotation with the arm at 90° of elevation. In the abduction movement the subject was facing the Kinect^{TM}. In the other movements, the subject was aside to the Kinect^{TM} with the arm that will make the movement closer to the Kinect^{TM}.

For the validation, this work required the participation of ten healthy subjects, six females and four males. During the acquisitions, the males wore shirts and the females fitting clothes. The lower body clothes were not relevant, but clothes with shiny surfaces, like belts, were avoided. In all movements, subjects were required to do three movements: the first with the arm at less than 90°, the second with the arm at approximately 90° and the last with the maximum achievable elevation.

4.2   Data Analysis

This work required the comparison between three different ROM measurement methods: the first using MotionPlux (frame rate of 800 Hz) the second and the third obtained with the Kinect^{TM} sensor (frame rate of 30 Hz). The Kinect^{TM} sensor was used to record joints' spatial coordinates provided by the official Microsoft Kinect^{TM} SDK and to record the depth frames. After computing the angles with each method, the Kinetic data was interpolated to achieve the same sampling frequency as MotionPlux. Then, a correlation with both data was done to synchronize them, ensuring that data would share a synchronous time reference.

Reference System. The MotionPlux system recorded the raw data and applied it a 1 Hz (empirically found) low pass Butterworth filter to reduce the influence of the dynamic acceleration. After this, the initial vector of the acceleration is saved and used as reference to measure the angles between this vector and the next vectors acquired. Thus, the result of this operation is a variation of the movement executed. For this reason, and because high rates influence triaxial accelerometer measurements [12], it was required that subjects remained stopped for 3 s in the initial and final positions.

The Kinect™ Skeleton Tracking. In order to study the Kinect™ Skeleton Tracking for rehabilitation purposes a short application to receive the information from the Kinect™ sensor was done. This application was developed in C# using the Visual Studio 2010 and the access of the data streams was made with the official drivers developed by Microsoft, the Microsoft Kinect™ SDK. With these drivers it is possible to use the Microsoft methods to access the anatomical landmarks. Thus, in the application the joints positions were found and shown in the stream of the RGB image with circles on the subject's joints.

In this work, only glenohumeral movements are analysed. The joints of interest to this study are the shoulder, elbow and wrist. For abduction, flexion and extension movements the shoulder and elbow positions are used. For internal and external rotation with the arm at 90 degrees of elevation the wrist position is used. To compute ROM measurements it was necessary to define two vectors and measure the angle between them. If the movement is abduction or flexion/extension, the first vector is composed by the shoulder and elbow spatial coordinates. Otherwise, the vector is composed by the elbow and wrist spatial coordinates. The second vector is used as reference.

Depth Analysis. The depth frames from the Kinect™ are recorded with the application mentioned before. The proposed algorithm can be divided in four main blocks. The first block is composed by the image processing techniques to obtain a binary image required for the remaining processing. The second block is used for identifying subject's movement and it is named automatic calibration. In the third block the anatomical landmarks are identified and in the fourth block the ROM measurements are computed. A flowchart that systematizes the processing main events is shown in Fig. 1.

The image processing techniques applied include a background subtraction to isolate the subject from the background, an opening (combination of a morphologic erosion followed by a dilation) to open up gaps between just-touching features and a morphological algorithm for boundaries extraction. The output of this block is a binary image with one single component, the subject.

The automatic calibration process is useful for recording some important measures of the subject and for detecting which movement the subject is doing. These measures are needed to find the shoulder, elbow and hand joint, as well as the head and the thorax inclination during any movement position.

In order to do this process, it is necessary to find the head position before the subject begins the movement. The head detection is done with the information of the vertical and horizontal projections of the binary image. As it can be seen in Fig. 2 the head y-coordinate is the first non-zero point in the horizontal projection. After detecting the head position, the algorithm is able to identify which

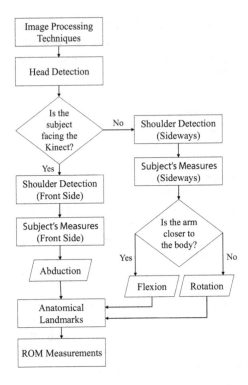

Fig. 1. Flowchart of the proposed algorithm

movement the subject does. The movement identification begins by detecting the subject position, i.e., determining if the subject is facing the Kinect^{TM} or aside to it. This detection is based on the differences between the left and the right horizontal projection of the binary image of half of the body. These projections are obtained dividing the subject's body by a vertical straight line that goes through the head position. Then, their differences are computed with the variance of the quotient between both projections. The variance is calculated with Eq. (1),

$$\sigma^2 = \frac{1}{N} \sum_{i=0}^{N} (x_i - \mu)^2 \quad , \quad x = \frac{P_1}{P_2} \tag{1}$$

where σ^2 is the population variance, N is the number of elements in the population, x_i is the i element from the population, μ is the population mean, P_1 is the horizontal projection of half of the body of the side on which the movement is executed (left or right) and P_2 is the other projection.

As it can be seen in Fig. 2 the general shape of the two projections when the subject is face to face with the Kinect^{TM} is similar. However, when the subject is aside to the Kinect^{TM} the differences are obvious. Therefore, the variance obtained when the subject is facing the Kinect^{TM} is smaller than the variance obtained in the other position. With the variance value it is possible to define

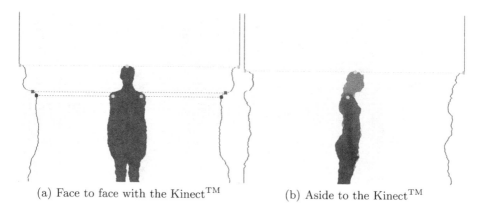

(a) Face to face with the Kinect^{TM} (b) Aside to the Kinect^{TM}

Fig. 2. Representation of the head and shoulders positions during the calibration process. In the left and right side of both images are also represented the half body horizontal projections

a threshold to distinguish both positions. Thus, if the position is the one represented in Fig. 2(a), the movement is abduction. Otherwise, it is necessary to decide between flexion/extension and internal/external rotation.

The next step is shoulders detection, that depends on subject's position. If the subject is doing an abduction movement, shoulders are detected calculating the maximum difference along the points of the horizontal projection (square in Fig. 2(a)). Once found this point, the first point where the difference is approximately constant is searched (circle in Fig. 2(a)). Thus, the shoulder position is composed by the x-coordinate of the square and the y-coordinate of the circle. In the other movements, the shoulder is detected based on the depth difference in the transition between the head and the remnant body. With the head and the shoulders detected, the measures presented in Fig. 3 begin to be recorded during approximately one second (30 frames). The measure chosen for the rest of the processing is the median of all measures. After this extraction, the subject receives the information that it can begin the movement. If the subject is in the position represented in Fig. 3(b), the algorithm starts to recognize which movement the subject is doing (flexion or rotation). The main difference between flexion/extension and internal/external rotation is the proximity of the arm with the body. Therefore, with the depth information provided by the Kinect^{TM}, an average with all depth values in the subject's body is calculated. Then, a depth threshold is established that is a percent of the depth average calculated before. If there is an object with a considerable area, near the head position and with the depth values smaller than the threshold, the movement is rotation. In flexion, almost the entire body has depth values greater than the threshold. During this process we extract the measures presented in Fig. 3.

To compute the angles achieved during the movements, a few anatomical landmarks need to be detected. This detection is done with the depth information provided by the Kinect^{TM} sensor combined with the horizontal and vertical

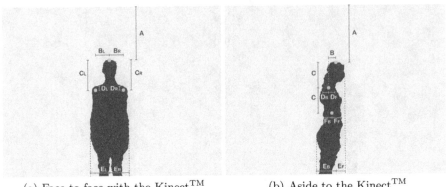

(a) Face to face with the Kinect^{TM} (b) Aside to the Kinect^{TM}

Fig. 3. Representation of the subject measures in two frames from the Kinect^{TM} after being processed

projections of the binary image. During processing it is necessary to first recognize the movement phase, because the way that the algorithm finds the anatomical landmarks depends on it. The movement phases are identified using the calibration measures. In Fig. 4 the different phases used for each movement are represented as well as the anatomical landmarks detected.

In the following points it is described how we find the anatomical landmarks during the movements.

- The **head** detection is done with the information of the maximums or extremes of the vertical or horizontal projection of the binary image. Depending on the movement phase, it can be necessary to remove arms' influence.
- The **thorax inclination** is calculated differently depending on the subject movement. In abduction and rotation the thorax inclination is computed by a linear regression based on several points in the centre of the subject's body. On the other hand, in flexion/extension the thorax inclination requires only a point in subject's body and the shoulder point. This point in the subject's body is found with the C measure from calibration (see Fig. 3(b)). In this movement we decided to use only one point because subject's arm complicates the measurements with several points.
- In abduction, the **shoulder** position is computed with the information of the thorax inclination combined with the distances from the calibration. Thus, the measures B and D from the calibration, Fig. 2(a), are predetermined by the thorax inclination. For flexion/extension, instead of using the thorax inclination, it is used the head position in combination with the calibration measures to find the shoulder. The shoulder is not required on internal/external rotation.
- Similarly with the head and depending on the movement phase, **hands** detection is done with the extremes of the vertical or horizontal projection. In flexion/extension, if the arm is overlaid with the body, the hand is not detected. However, in rotation movement, even if the arm is overlaid with the body, the

hand position is detected based on the forearm length obtained during other movement phases.

- Finally, in abduction and flexion/extension movements, each **elbow** is computed assuming that the humerus length corresponds to 40 % of the distance between the shoulder and the extremity of the hand [13]. In rotation, the approximate elbow position is calculated with the calibration measures of the shoulder, because in this movement the subject's arm is at 90° of abduction. Therefore, the shoulder coordinates are approximately the same of the elbow.

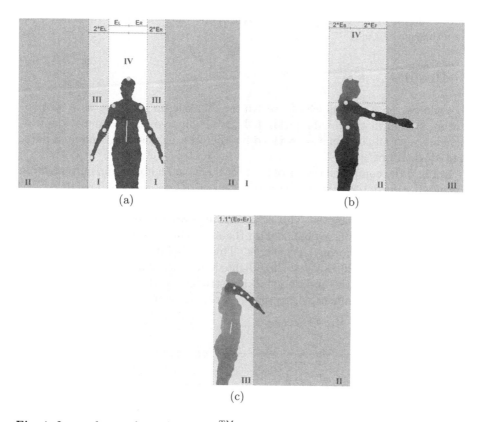

Fig. 4. Image frames from the Kinect™ sensor after being processed and with the movement phases and anatomical landmarks represented. (a) Abduction movement in phase I; (b) Flexion movement in phase III; (c) Internal rotation in phase II

After this detection process, the ROM measurements can be finally calculated. The way that ROM measurements are done depends on the movement performed. In abduction and flexion/extension the procedures are the same. However, as the detection of the anatomical landmarks in internal/external rotation is not precise, it was necessary to find another way to compute it. In abduction and flexion/extension the ROM measurements are computed in millimetres and in a 3D coordinates system. Similarly with the Kinect[TM] Skeleton Tracking method, it is necessary to define two vectors for measuring the angle between them. With our algorithm it is possible to use the thorax inclination as reference instead of the world reference. For internal/external rotation, ROM measurements are computed in pixels and in 2D coordinates. This decision was made because the rotation detection is done with the forearm position and if the forearm is not perpendicular to the arm, the rotation is not influenced. Therefore, the z coordinate information would influence the measurement wrongly. Thus, in this movement, one vector is a linear regression calculated with the shortest depth values in the subject's forearm and the other is the reference that the user wants to use.

5   Results

To evaluate the performance of the Kinect[TM] Skeleton Tracking as a motion capture system in the rehabilitation field, we compared the computed data of the joints' spatial coordinates provided by Microsoft against the computed data from MotionPlux.

In Fig. 5 the computed data from both systems in an abduction movement is presented. After interpolation and correlation of the signals it is possible to see that their general shape is identical. However, the differences between the signals increase with higher angles. This situation also occurs in flexion movement. Those differences can be explained with the instability of the shoulders position when the subject performs large angles. This instability can be seen in Fig. 6 where the troubling instants are highlighted in grey. During the acquisitions it was observed that the skeleton tracking struggles with objects in the scene. Therefore, the environment where the acquisitions are made can be a problem in clinical uses.

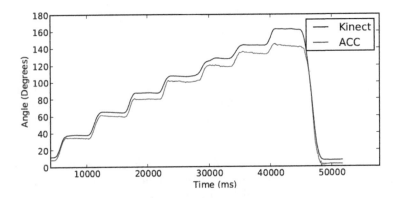

Fig. 5. Representation of the computed data from the Kinect[TM] Skeleton Tracking and the MotionPlux in an abduction movement

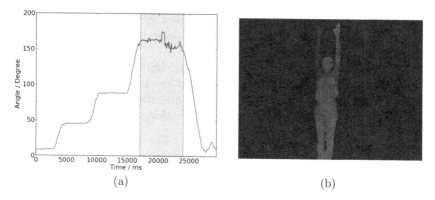

(a)   (b)

Fig. 6. (a) Representation of the angles executed during an abduction movement with the troubling instants highlighted in grey; (b) Depth frame acquired in one of these troubling instants

The accuracy of the Kinect^{TM} Skeleton Tracking and the proposed algorithm was calculated using the Mean Error (ME) and the Standard Deviation (SD). In Table 1 the comparison between both methods and the reference system are shown. All results were obtained with variations of the initial and final positions instead of the maximum angle recorded.

Table 1. Comparison between the Kinect^{TM} Skeleton Tracking and the proposed algorithm based on depth analysis

Movement	The Kinect^{TM} Skeleton Tracking		Depth Analysis	
	ME/°	SD/°	ME/°	SD/°
Abduction	2.91	2.51	1.14	1.39
Flexion	13.13	17.11	1.23	1.53
Rotation	18.02	19.34	1.23	1.47

As it can be seen in Table 1, the Kinect^{TM} Skeleton Tracking has a ME higher than the proposed algorithm in all movements studied. However, in abduction the differences obtained with both methods are not as relevant as in the other movements. Only in this movement, we consider that the Kinect^{TM} Skeleton Tracking can be used to do ROM measurements in the rehabilitation field. The other movements presented ME higher than 10 degrees. Therefore, these ROM measurements cannot be used to do accurate ROM measurements. The difficulties with the ROM measurements in flexion/extension and internal/external rotation were essentially due to the fact that the subject is aside to the Kinect^{TM} in these movements. Thus, the tracking is more difficult since some body parts are occluded from the camera. If the subject is facing the Kinect[TM] in these movements, the problems remain because in certain movement phases the arm is perpendicular to the Kinect[TM] occluding the joints of interest.

The proposed algorithm presented lower ME than the Kinect[TM] Skeleton Tracking. In all studied movements the ME was less than 1.5°. So, in the aside movements our algorithm improved an order of magnitude when compared with the same results from the Kinect[TM] Skeleton Tracking (See Table 1).

6   Discussion

Biofeedback is a useful addition in the rehabilitation field. It can improve the performance of the training allowing the patient and the therapist to know the patient's evolution in real-time. This knowledge in real-time is a tool to adapt current training to the patient's needs. An interactive system able to show patient's evolution might also draw additional motivation that can be translated in a more effective training.

The proposed algorithm has the advantage of being a ROM measurements system and a biofeedback system. Therefore, our system can substitute the goniometer, which is the most common tool used in the clinics to do ROM measurements, bringing the innovation of a biofeedback system. With the goniometer the measures are done manually. Therefore, it is not practical and its results present a 5–10° error [9]. On the other hand, our method is done in real-time, it is an non-intrusive, easy to use system with an accuracy less than 1.5° in all movements studied. The ROM measurements with the proposed algorithm also have the advantage of measuring thorax inclination. Thus, it is possible to adjust the calculation of the shoulder angle with the thorax inclination. If the subject tilts the body because it makes it easier to achieve a higher angle, ROM measurements will not increase because of that. With the biofeedback system the subject can also be prevented from compensating with the body, improving this way the effectiveness of his exercise.

The accuracy of the proposed algorithm showed that it is able to overcome the limitations associated with the Kinect[TM] Skeleton Tracking provided by Microsoft. This algorithm has several advantages in applications where accuracy is not required or the general trends in the movement are sufficient. In abduction, the mean error of 2.91° was considered acceptable for ROM measurements. In the flexion/extension and internal/external rotation the mean error was higher than 10°. Therefore, the goniometer is able to do ROM measurements with higher accuracy, being preferable for this task. As the Microsoft Kinect[TM] SDK is proprietary and closed source, it is not possible to adapt it to our needs nor extend it or improve its abilities. For this reason, our algorithm is limited to the use of the depth map information.

Although the developed algorithm presents an accurate way to do ROM measurements, it also has some disadvantages when compared with the Kinect[TM] Skeleton Tracking. As we are working directly with the depth information, our algorithm is limited to the movements studied in the glenohumeral joint. However, we plan to extend it to other body parts applying the same principles used in this work. The environment is a limitation for both methods. Although the Kinect™ Skeleton Tracking does not require a static environment, it was verified that it struggles with objects in the scene. On the other hand, as the background subtraction is done in our algorithm, the objects in the scene are not a problem for it. However, optimal results are not achieved without a static background.

7   Conclusions and Future Work

In conclusion, the Kinect sensor in combination with biofeedback techniques can represent a breakthrough in the rehabilitation field. The proposed algorithm and the Kinect Skeleton Tracking can be used in this clinical area for different applications. The Kinect Skeleton Tracking is useful for applications, like counting repetitions, where the general trends in the movement are sufficient. On the other hand, if more accurate measures are required, the proposed algorithm is able to overcome the limitations of the Kinect Skeleton Tracking.

For future work we plan to do a further validation and introduce our ROM measurements in an electromyographic biofeedback system. Once the patients with muscular abnormality normally have problems with their ROM, it would be relevant to introduce a new biofeedback protocol to use, at the same time, the ROM and EMG information. A more exhaustive validation with subjects with any muscular pain should also be done, to prove that their possible body differences were not influencing the precision of the proposed algorithm.

References

1. Lünenburger, L., Colombo, G., Riener, R.: Biofeedback for robotic gait rehabilitation. J. NeuroEng. Rehabil. **4**(1), 1 (2007)
2. Begg, R., Palaniswami, M.: Computational Intelligence for Movement Sciences: Neural Networks and Other Emerging Techniques. Idea Group Publishing, Hershey (2006)
3. Dutta, T.: Evaluation of the kinect sensor for 3-D kinematic measurement in the workplace. Appl. Ergon. **43**, 645–649 (2011)
4. Pece, F., Kautz, J., Weyrich, T.: Three depth-camera technologies compared. In: Engineering in Medicine and Biology Society, pp. 1188–1193 (2012)
5. Kourosh Khoshelham and Sander Oude Elberink: Accuracy and resolution of kinect depth data for indoor mapping applications. Sensors **12**(2), 1437–1454 (2012)
6. Clark, R.A., Pua, Y.-H., Fortin, K., Ritchie, C., Webster, K.E., Denehy, L., Bryant, A.L.: Validity of the microsoft kinect for assessment of postural control. Gait & Posture **36**(3), 372–377 (2012)
7. Obdržálek, Š., Kurillo, G., Ofli, F., Bajcsy, R., Seto, E., Jimison, H., Pavel, M.: Accuracy and robustness of kinect pose estimation in the context of coaching of elderly population. In: Engineering in Medicine and Biology Society, pp. 1188–1193 (2012)
8. Fernández-Baena, A., Susin, A., Lligadas, X.: Biomechanical validation of upper-body and lower-body joint movements of kinect motion capture data for rehabilitation treatments. In: 2012 4th International Conference on Intelligent Networking and Collaborative Systems (INCoS), pp. 656–661. IEEE (2012)

9. Kitsunezaki, N., Adachi, E., Masuda, T., Mizusawa, J.: Kinect applications for the physical rehabilitation. In: 2013 IEEE International Symposium on Medical Measurements and Applications Proceedings (MeMeA), pp. 294–299. IEEE (2013)
10. Metsis, V., Jangyodsuk, P., Athitsos, V., Iversen, M., Makedon, F.: Computer aided rehabilitation for patients with rheumatoid arthritis. In: 2013 International Conference on Computing, Networking and Communications (ICNC), pp. 97–102. IEEE (2013)
11. Beckert, J., Silva, F., Palma, S.: Inter-rater reliability of the visual estimation of shoulder abduction angles and the agreement of measurements with an accelerometer. In: Proceedings of ECSS2009, Oslo, Norway (2009)
12. Bernmark, E., Wiktorin, C.: A triaxial accelerometer for measuring arm movements. Appl. Ergon. **33**(6), 541–547 (2002)
13. Loomis, A.: Figure Drawing for All It's Worth. Penguin Group (USA) Incorporated, New York (1943)

Online Classifier Adaptation for the Detection of P300 Target Recognition Processes in a Complex Teleoperation Scenario

Hendrik Woehrle[1]([✉]) and Elsa Andrea Kirchner[1,2]

[1] Robotics Innovation Center, German Research Center
for Artificial Intelligence (DFKI GmbH),
Robert-Hooke-Str. 1, Bremen, Germany
hendrik.woehrle@dfki.de
[2] Universität Bremen, Arbeitsgruppe Robotik,
Robert-Hooke-Str. 1, Bremen, Germany

Abstract. The detection of event related potentials and their usage for innovative applications became an increasingly important research topic for brain computer interfaces in the last couple of years. However, brain computer interfaces use methods that need to be trained on subject-specific data before they can be used. This problem must be solved for real-world applications in which humans are multi tasking and hence are to some degree are less predictable in their behavior compared to classical set ups for brain computer interfacing. In this paper, we show the detection and passive usage of the P300 related brain activity in a highly uncontrolled and noisy application scenario. The subjects are multi tasking, i.e., they perform a demanding senso-motor task, i.e., the telemanipulate a real robotic arm while responding to important messages. For telemanipulation, the subject wears an active exoskeleton to control a robotic arm, which is presented to him in a virtual scenario. By online analysis of the subject's electroencephalogram we detect P300 related target recognition processes to infer on upcoming response behavior on presented task-relevant messages (Targets) or missing of response behavior in case a Target was not recognized. We show that a classifier that is trained to distinguish between brain activity evoked by recognized task-relevant stimuli (recognized Targets) and ignored frequent task-irrelevant stimuli (Standards) can be applied to classify between brain activity evoked by recognized targets and brain activity that is evoked in case that task-relevant stimuli are *not* recognized (Missed Targets). The applied transfer of classifier results in reduced performance. We show that this draw back of the approach can strongly be improved by using online machine learning tools to adapt the pre-trained classifier to the new class, i.e., to the Missed Target class, that was not used during training of the classifier.

Keywords: Brain computer interfaces · Embedded brain reading · P300 · Single trial detection · Exoskeleton · Adaptation

© Springer-Verlag Berlin Heidelberg 2014
H.P. da Silva et al. (Eds.): PhyCS 2014, LNCS 8908, pp. 105–118, 2014.
DOI: 10.1007/978-3-662-45686-6_7

1   Introduction

Online-analysis and detection of specific patterns in electroencephalographic (EEG) data has been used for various applications, e.g., brain computer interfaces (BCIs). Current EEG-based BCIs are using classification and data dependent signal processing methods to detect specific patterns in EEG. They highly depend on *training data* that has to be used for the calibration of the system before they can be used to detect the patterns in the *application data*. Usually, the training data has to be *subject-specific*, i.e., it has to be acquired from the subject in training sessions directly before the usage of the system. Further, the recorded data should be *clean*, i.e., free of artifacts that might affect the training or detection process, as well as *task-specific*, i.e., must consist of data that is directly related to the patterns that are supposed to be detected. Therefore, most results are conducted in highly controlled artificial scenarios, where most of the possible disturbance sources have been excluded by experimental design and the subject may even be fixed in a specific position.

For many applications this is no drawback, especially if BCIs are applied as active interfaces, i.e., to control a machine or computer [2,5,17,20,25]. If, however, the patterns that should be detected in the brain activity are no longer actively produced, as it is the case for passive BCIs [4,26], then background EEG that is evoked by the active task may overlay with the relevant brain activity. Since the subject is possibly performing multiple and changing tasks, the background EEG may differ strongly depending on the situation and performed active task or action of the user and thus affects the training data. For future practical applications of passive approaches [4,6,10,11,26], it is required to expose the systems and subjects to concrete, realistic use-cases, that are more uncontrolled and performed in perturbed environments. These conditions likely increase the amount of noise in the training as well as application data and may therefore impair the detection accuracy.

A further problem exists, if the amount of training data is small. It might not be possible to acquire a large amount of training examples in complex application scenarios, in which the relevant class (like the missing of an event) might strongly be underrepresented. This is a general problem, since the detection accuracy of data-dependent signal processing and classification methods depends on the amount of available training data. Hence, approaches that can handle a reduced amount of training examples must be developed and applied.

One approach that can be applied in this case is the transfer of pre-trained classifiers between different sessions. For example, a classifier can be pre-trained on data that, e.g., has previously been acquired in another session and is reused for the actual session. Such classifier transfer [18] could further be shown to perform well for a transfer of classifier between tasks in which the same event related activity has to be detected [7] or between similar types of event related potentials (ERPs) like different types of error potentials [8]. In a recent work we showed that the transfer of classifier is also possible between classes that "miss" a pronounced pattern, i.e., the P300 [13]. Hence, the data processing methods (classifiers and spatial filters) need not to be trained and tested on examples that are evoked by the same brain processes, like same or similar error detection processes, but by brain processes that evoke brain pattern, which are similar in shape and characteristics, i.e., miss a prominent ERP or pattern of ERPs.

Unfortunately, any transfer of classifier results in a drop of the classification accuracy, i.e., an increase of the number of wrong predictions that are made by such a classifier. However, if the classifier is adapted by examples of the new (former unknown) class using data that is acquired while it is in use, i.e., during its application, it is possible to compensate this draw back of the classifier transfer approach to a certain amount.

By now, our investigations have been conducted in controlled experimental setups in an offline fashion. In this paper, we investigate the ability to detect the P300 ERP in a demanding dual-task application scenario that combines an oddball paradigm with a second task. We show that the detection of P300 related target recognition processes and even more important the *missing* of target recognition processes can be performed online while a subject is performing a demanding and realistic interaction task that occupies the operators attention. This task consists of the teleoperation of a real robotic arm through a labyrinth via a virtual immersion scenario.

The paper makes the following contributions: (1) we demonstrate that the online, single trial detection of the P300 potential is possible in an application scenario that is affected by a high number of noise sources and artifacts and requires dual task performance from the subject [12], i.e., distracts the subject from the perception of task relevant stimuli; (2) we show that the few number of examples of training data of a specific class can be compensated to a certain degree by classifier transfer. (3) we show that the adaptation of the classifier is helpful if it is transferred between sessions under certain circumstances.

2   Application Scenario

In the proposed application scenario, we investigate whether it is possible to reliably detect target recognition processes as well as the missing of target recognition processes while a subject is performing a demanding teleoperation task.

Precisely, the experimental setup was as follows (see Fig. 1A): The subjects were wearing an exoskeleton that covered their back and right arm [3], and a smart glove on their hand that were used as input devices for the teleoperation task.

In addition, participants were equipped with a head mounted display (HMD) on which the teleoperation site (including surroundings, labyrinth and robot) could be seen in 3D.

Additionally to the 3D environment, information from the control system, a camera picture of the real scene and tools like a gyroscope depicting the orientation of the end-effector were at any time in the operators field of view. Head and hand movements of the operator were tracked (InterSense, Billerica, USA) and used to update the HMD.

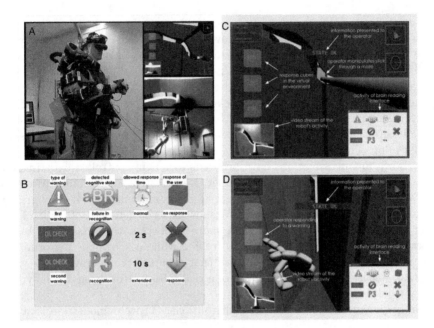

Fig. 1. Teleoperation scenario and operator monitoring system.

The subjects had two main tasks that had to be performed at the same time: (a) to control a robotic arm (*teleoperation task*) using the exoskeleton, and (b) to respond to specific messages (*oddball task*).

2.1 The Teleoperation Task

In the teleoperation task, the end-effector of a robotic arm had to be steered through a labyrinth (see Fig. 1C). This task is similar to a wire loop game, i.e., a certain path has to be followed and touching the labyrinth had to be avoided. The movements of the robotic arm were controlled via the exoskeleton by mapping the state and relative position of the exoskeleton components to a Mitubishi PA-10 robotic arm (see Fig. 1A in the lower right corner) via a virtual model (see Fig. 1A in the upper right corner) thereof (depending on the concrete type of investigation, see Sect. 3).

The teleoperation task is difficult and demanding for the subject, and therefore forces the subject to concentrate on it. Further, the subject was requested to rest from time to time. In each run 24 ± 8 rest periods had to be performed [23]. During rest the active exoskeleton kept the operators arm in position. While this was the case the operator was not allowed to respond to any warning (infrequent task relevant stimuli, see below) that were presented to him in an oddball fashion throughout the run.

2.2   The Oddball Task

In the oddball-task, the subject had to respond to infrequent *task relevant* stimuli (*"Targets"*, see Fig. 2B) by touching one of three virtual cubes that were integrated into the virtual scenario as response targets for answering specific messages in a certain time frame (see Fig. 1D). Besides the task relevant messages also frequent task irrelevant messages (*"Standards"*, see Fig. 2A) were presented to the operator but required no response. Due to the oddball design [19], i.e., the presentation of infrequent task relevant stimuli mixed with frequent task irrelevant stimuli, it was expected that P300 related brain processes [9,12,16,19,22] will be evoked in case of recognized infrequent task relevant messages but not in case of frequent task irrelevant messages or task relevant but *not* recognized, i.e., missed, task relevant messages (*"Missed Targets"*). In recorded training data it was determined whether a Target was recognized or not by the occurrence or missing of a response 10 s after a Target stimulus was presented.

2.3   The Operator Monitoring System

To support the operator in the scenario, an operator monitoring system (OMS) [11] was included into the setup. The purpose of the OMS was to monitor the operators cognitive state and the current state of scenario in order to adjust the course of events that were shown to the operator to minimize distraction of the operator and optimize her or his support by appropriate scheduling of messages.

The allowed response time was 2 s in case that target recognition processes could *not* be detected after a Target was presented (in case of *Missed Target*, see Fig. 1B, first warning for "oil check" was missed) or to extend the allowed response time to 10 s in case target recognition process were detected after a Target was presented and recognized (in case of *Target*, see Fig. 1B, second warning for "oil check" was recognized).

By adapting the allowed response time in this manner allows to give the operator a longer time for responses in case he recognized the warning, which was especially relevant in case that the operator was in a rest position and was not able to respond. On the other hand a task relevant message could be repeated rather quick in case that target recognition processes could not be detected after a Target message was presented.

To enable this adjustment of the virtual scenario by the OMS, we used machine learning techniques to detect the P300 ERP in the subjects EEG. Therefore, a classifier had to be trained to distinguish examples of the class *Target* from examples of the class *Missed Targets* online. Since the operators were highly trained in the scenario they usually miss only a few Target messages, hence the amount of Missed Target examples that could be recorded was very low. Thus, we used EEG activity evoked by irrelevant Standard messages instead of EEG activity evoked by Missed Target messages during the training phase of the data processing to later distinguish between Targets and Missed Targets.

2.4   Visual Stimuli in the Operator Monitoring System

The stimuli shown to the operator are illustrated in Fig. 2. (A) The frequently shown *Standard* marker has the text *STATE OK*. (B) One of the three possible *Targets*. The possibilities are *MAN ENTERED*, *OIL TEMPERATURE* or *COM REQUEST*. (C) The operators response must be related to the warning. In this case, it is the cube with the label *COM*. In case of a correct response, it is highlighted in green. (D) If the operator did not respond in time, a repeated and highlighted second *Target* is shown. (E) If the operator did not respond to the second Target in time, a third obtrusive error message is shown. (F) In any case it might happen that the operator touches a cube with a label that does not correspond to the shown Target. In this case, the cube is highlighted in red.

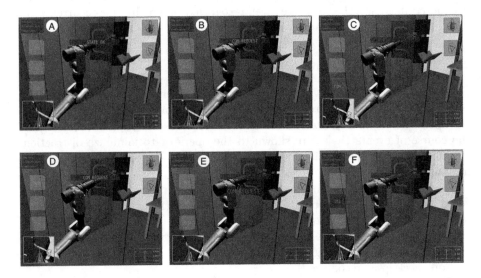

Fig. 2. The warnings and responses shown in the virtual immersion teleoperation operator monitoring scenario (Color figure online).

3   Methods and Experimental Procedures

The experiments were performed with three male subjects (age 27.33 ± 2.52), with a total of ten recording sessions.

3.1   Setup and Data Acquisition

The data was acquired with a 64-channel actiCap system and two amplifiers (both from Brainproducts, Munich, Germany) at 5 kHz sampling rate. Four electrodes (FC5, FC6, FT7, FT8) of the extended 10–20 system were omitted to allow the HMD to be mounted. Thus, 60 channels were used for the recording.

The actual prediction system was active in four of ten sessions (online runs) and inactive in six out of ten sessions. Thus, the overall data consisted of 4 online and 6 pseudo-online sessions. Pseudo-online sessions consisted of three, and online sessions of four runs, with the forth run being the actual online run. Otherwise they were treated in the same way. A single run lasted in average about 13.64 ± 3.85 min.

The data acquired in the last run of each session was used for evaluation of our system, and the other sessions for training of the system. The pseudo-online sessions were analyzed offline after the experiments and are used here to provide a more comprehensive data basis.

The runs contained between 466 and 1553 (in average ≈ 865) *Standards*, between 16 and 51 (in average ≈ 35) *Targets*, and between 1 and 54 (in average ≈ 8) *Missed Targets*.

All processing was performed on equally-shaped windows of data with 1 s of duration, which were cut-out and labeled according to the occurrence of a *Standard*, *Target* or *Missed Target*.

Between two runs there was a short break of 2–3 min, except before the last run in the online sessions where the movement prediction system had to be trained and thus the break lasted around 10 min.

3.2   Processing Methods

We used our software pySPACE (Signal Processing And Classification Environment) [14, 15][1] for online and pseudo-online data analysis.

All windows were processed independently from each other. The data was preprocessed in several steps in order to extract the relevant features for the classifier. First, the data was standardized channel-wise by subtracting the mean signal value of the channel and divided by the standard deviation of the channel in the corresponding signal window. Next, a decimation with an anti-alias finite impulse response filter was performed to reduce the sampling rate of the data from 5 kHz to 25 Hz. This was followed by another band pass filter with pass band from 0.1 to 4.0 Hz.

Afterwards, the dimension of the data was reduced further in several steps. First, the xDAWN spatial filter [21] was applied to reduce the 60 channels data to eight channels. The xDAWN spatial filter splits the data in noise and signal-plus-noise subspaces to, at the same time, extract meaningful signal information and reduce the dimension of the data. The number of eight channels was chosen based on previous experience with other experimental setups.

We used straight lines, a special form of local polynomial features, as features for the classifier. The straight lines were fit channel-wise to segments of the data. Each segment lasted for about 400 ms and adjacent segments overlapped by about 400 ms. The slope of the lines were used as features. These were standardized again in the next processing step.

---

[1] Available at http://pyspace.github.com/pyspace.

3.3   Classification and Adaptation

As described in Sect. 1, a common problem is the dependency of the applied data processing methods on training data.

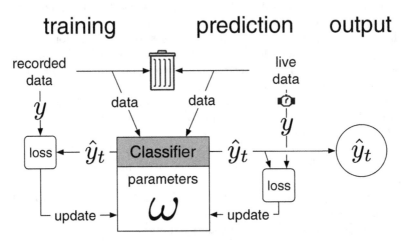

Fig. 3. Training, adaptation and usage of the classifier: In the *training phase*, a classifier is first trained on recorded datasets to compute the corresponding parameter vector w. These can be recorded either directly in training data sessions or previously stored data is used. Afterwards it can be used to perform *predictions* $\hat{y}$ on live data. If an adaptable classifier is used, the classifier can be *updated* with new data and labels (which are generated by the subjects behavior in the application).

Our strategy to adapt the classifier in the application is depicted in Fig. 3. Depending on the events that happen in the application, the classifier performs a prediction (e.g. if a Target is shown, the corresponding window of EEG data is classified whether it is perceived as a Target or not). The result is sent to the OMS environment and the allowed reaction times are adjusted (see Sect. 2.4).

Afterwards, the *correct* label is inferred based on the reaction of the subject in the application:

- if the subject responds to the Target, we assume that it has perceived the stimulus and adapt the classifier with the new data labeled as *Target*
- if the subject does not respond tho the Target, we assume that the subject *missed* the Target and therefore adapt the classifier with the new data labeled as *Standard* (TM case)
- in the case that a Standard was shown, no reaction of the subject is required and we adapt the classifier with the new data labeled as *Standard* (TS case).

This continuous adaptation process requires a classifier that can easily be adapted with the new data-label pair. Most Standard *batch* classification algorithms require the whole training data set to be available for the training of classifier and require extensive computations in the training process. This is a major problem for the online adaptation as it is performed in our application, since the classifier is frequently updated. Therefore, we investigate and compare two different strategies for the classification and adaptation.

As a reference, we used an *unadaptive* soft-margin support vector machine (SVM) with a linear kernel for classification. The SVM is a frequently applied classifier that gives the baseline. The complexity regularization hyperparameter was optimized using a grid search (tested values: $10^{-6}, 10^{-5}, \ldots, 10^{0}$) and an internal 5-fold cross validation. Only the data acquired in the training runs (see Sect. 3.1) were used for the preliminary training and hyperparameter optimization.

An approach that can be applied here is the usage of *online* classification algorithms. Popular online classification algorithm are the passive aggressive perceptron (PAP) algorithms [1]. The PAPs have an analogous approach to the SVM, since both try to separate the two classes by constructing a separating hyperplane with a maximum margin by minimizing the hinge loss $\ell_h(y_t, \hat{y}_t) = max\{0, 1 - y\hat{y}_t\}$, where the linear prediction model is given by $\hat{y}_t = \mathbf{w}_t^T \mathbf{x}_t$ (see Eq. 1). Different variations of PAPs exist, we discuss the PA1 perceptron in the following, which has the closest similarity to a soft-margin support vector machine.

The update rule for the PA1 perceptron is given in Eq. 1.

$$\mathbf{w}_{t+1} = \mathbf{w}_t + \min\left\{C, \frac{\ell_h(\mathbf{w}_t^T \mathbf{x}_t, y_t)}{||\mathbf{x}_t||^2}\right\} y_t \mathbf{x}_t \tag{1}$$

Here, $\mathbf{w}_t$ denotes the classification parameter vector at *time t*, i.e. before the updated has been performed, $\mathbf{x}_t$ denote the data for time t and y_t the corresponding label. The employed loss function ℓ_h is the hinge loss. The PA1 perceptron incorporates an *aggressiveness parameter* C that controls the aggressiveness of the update, which can improve the generalization ability of the obtained classifiers in the presence of noise.

The update requires only a minimum of computations, which makes the PA1 perceptron a promising target method for the online adaptation. However, they are not commonly used in BCIs and therefore require investigation how they compare to *standard* algorithms, like the SVM.

3.4   Evaluation

The data was evaluated with respect to the ability of a classifier to

1. distinguish online and in single trial between EEG examples that contain patterns related to target recognition processes (that evoke a P300) and EEG examples that miss these patterns, and
2. be adaptable for the online classification
3. regarding differences between the SVM and the different PAP variants.

We expect that both, Missed Targets and Standards would not evoke P300 related patterns while Targets do. Since enough training data was available we first analyzed how well a classifier trained on *Standard* and *Target* examples performs to distinguish between both classes (Target vs. Standard (TS) case).

Afterwards, we used a classifier that was trained on *Standard* and *Target* examples to distinguish between *Target* and *Missed Target* examples (Target vs. Missed (TM) case) which was the relevant application case (see Sect. 2). To compare both results allows us to estimate how well the classifier transfer performs in a demanding application teleoperation scenario.

Furthermore, we investigate the transfer between sessions. That is, the classifier and all other data dependent methods are *trained* on a specific session, and afterwards *tested* on all other recorded sessions of the *same* subject. This is an important application case, since usually the acquisition of training data sets is time consuming and exhausting for the subject. The avoidance of training data recording sessions is even more important in complex setups like the one that is presented in Sect. 2, since the maintenance and handling of multiple elaborate (e.g. exoskelettons and virtual immersion setups) increase the effort by a large amount.

4   Results and Discussion

For the evaluation of the classification performance we use the Balanced Accuracy (BA), which is given by $\frac{1}{2}TPR + \frac{1}{2}TNR$, where TPR and TNR are the true positive and true negative rate, respectively. Accordingly, a BA score of 0.5 corresponds to random guessing, while a BA score of 1.0 would correspond to a *perfect* classifier. The BA is not affected by an unbalanced number of examples in each class, as it is the case here [24].

The obtained classification performance (as BA) for the different runs and sessions in the normal (intra session) case is shown in Table 1. The results correspond to the *single trial* detection of the P300 ERP.

Table 1. Classification performance for Target vs. Standard (TS case) and Target vs. Missed Targets (TM case) for the SVM and PA1 perceptron (PA) in the normal case: the corresponding classifier is trained on the training data sets that were directly recorded before the test session. The PA1 perceptron is either used unadaptive (UA) or adaptive (A). The first 6 columns on the left contain the results for the *pseudo-online* sessions, the 4 columns on the right contain the results for the *online* sessions.

Evaluation	S1 R1	S1 R2	S2 R1	S2 R2	S3 R1	S3 R2	S1 R_{ol}1	S1 R_{ol}2	S1 R_{ol}3	S2 R_{ol}1
TS SVM	0.84	0.97	0.96	0.95	0.88	0.86	0.91	0.88	0.85	0.93
TM SVM	0.64	0.98	0.86	0.72	0.83	0.78	0.81	0.9	0.80	0.94
TS PA UA	0.79	0.94	0.96	0.94	0.86	0.83	0.86	0.86	0.85	0.90
TM PA UA	0.71	0.97	0.86	0.82	0.82	0.77	0.88	0.88	0.88	0.84
TS PA A	0.82	0.91	0.94	0.94	0.86	0.80	0.84	0.88	0.85	0.93
TM PA A	0.63	0.98	0.80	0.72	0.86	0.64	0.7	0.96	0.73	0.74

The average classification performance (as BA) in the TM case of the SVM is 0.827 ± 0.103, which is slightly lower than in the TS case of the SVM (0.902 ± 0.048). It can be observed that in 8 of 10 sessions the difference of the BA is 0.1 or less, and in 5 of 10 sessions it is even 0.05 or less.

The average classification performances of the PA1 perceptron in the TS case are 0.88 ± 0.06 (without adaptation) and 0.87 ± 0.05 (with adaptation). If the PA1 perceptron is used in the TM case, the average classification performances decrease to 0.84 ± 0.07 (without adaptation) and 0.78 ± 0.13 (with adaptation).

This shows that the achieved classification performance of our system works well for the P300 single trial detection for both the TM and TS cases despite the disturbance-prone setup. In addition, there is no remarkable difference between the TM and TS cases.

Furthermore, the difference between the BA score in the pseudo-online and online sessions is negligible (average classification performance TS case pseudo-online: $\approx 0.9089 \pm 0.057$, online: $\approx 0.893 \pm 0.037$; TM case pseudo-online: $\approx 0.803 \pm 0.110$, online $\approx 0.864 \pm 0.070$).

Furthermore, only small differences of the classification performance between SVM and PA1 perceptron can be observed in the unadaptive case.

An unexpected result is the decrease of the classification performance if the adaptive PA1 perceptron is used. This result can also be observed in the inter-session transfer (see below).

Table 2. Classification performance for Target vs. Standard (TS case) and Target vs. Missed Targets (TM case) of the PA1 perceptron (PA) for the session transfer. The PA1 perceptron is either used unadaptive (UA) or adaptive (A). We report the average performances for each recording session as training data vs. all other recording session of the same subject as test sessions.

Evaluation	S1 R1	S1 R2	S2 R1	S2 R2	S3 R1	S3 R2	S1 $R_{ol}1$	S1 $R_{ol}2$	S1 $R_{ol}3$	S2 $R_{ol}1$
TS PA UA	0.77	0.84	0.95	0.86	0.82	0.84	0.82	0.81	0.83	0.88
TM PA UA	0.82	0.82	0.77	0.81	0.64	0.75	0.80	0.78	0.89	0.78
TS PA A	0.83	0.83	0.94	0.90	0.78	0.80	0.85	0.84	0.84	0.89
TM PA A	0.72	0.72	0.78	0.73	0.72	0.73	0.72	0.70	0.81	0.74

However, if we perform an inter-session transfer, we can observe a general decrease of the classification performance in the TS case, e.g. for the unadaptive PA1 perceptron to 0.837 ± 0.049, as shown in Table 2. However, this decrease can be compensated by a certain amount if the PA1 perceptron is adapted in the application (a classification performance of 0.849 ± 0.042 is achieved). An improvement of the classification performance in this case is an expectable result.

In the TM case we observe again a decrease of the classification performance, too (0.81 ± 0.084), and furthermore a decrease of the classification performance for in the adaptive case (0.732 ± 0.095).

The decrease of the classification performance for the transfer between sessions is reasonable and has been observed in other investigations before. An unexpected result was the unability to compensate the decrease of the classification performance if an adaptive classifier was used.

Especially in the case that the PA1 classifier was adapted with Missed Targets in the TM case resulted in a decrease of the classification performance instead of an improvement. We assume the following reasons for this result:

1. Differences in the neurophysiological properties between Missed Targets and Standards. It has been shown in [13], that such differences exist. We assume that this has a negative impact on the adaptation of the classifier, since it was originally *not* trained with samples that belong to the Missed Targets category.
2. Changes in the ratio of the amounts of the different classes. Standards occur very frequently, while Missed Targets only occur occasionally. This again is a change of the properties compared to the original training data which might have a negative impact on the classification performance.

5   Conclusions and Future Work

The presented results show that it is possible to detect the P300 in a complex and noisy application scenario where the operator of a robot has to perform a dual task, i.e., to teleoperate a robot and to respond to warnings. Furthermore, our results show that a classifier can be transferred between classes in case that both classes, here Standard and Missed Targets, that miss a prominent pattern in the EEG signal, here the P300 ERP. This transfer works for most cases very well with only a small decrease of the classification performance. However, online adaptation of the classifier during the application of only the classifier helps to reduce this decrease by a certain amount.

In some cases the performance does decrease by a larger amount in the TM case. Causes for this have to be investigated.

In future, we plan to improve the signal processing and pattern recognition methodology further to reduce the amount of required training data and to compensate for changes of the user itself, like fatigue. Since usually adaptive methods have a positive impact on the classification performance, we assume that the usage of more sophisticated methods should also be helpful for complex application scenarios like the one presented here. However, the reasons why this is not the case here have to be investigated.

In addition, we plan to use and evaluate our system in even more advanced and complex application scenarios, e.g., the supervision of operators that control several robots simultaneously.

Acknowledgements. This work was funded by the *Federal Ministry of Economics and Technology* (BMWi, grant no. 50 RA 1012 and 50 RA 1011).

References

1. Crammer, K., Dekel, O., Keshet, J., Shalev-Shwartz, S., Singer, Y.: Online passive-aggressive algorithms. J. Mach. Learn. Res. **7**, 551–585 (2006)
2. Farwell, L.A., Donchin, E.: Talking off the top of your head: toward a mental prosthesis utilizing event-related brain potentials. Electroencephalogr. Clin. Neurophysiol. **70**(6), 510–523 (1988)
3. Folgheraiter, M., Jordan, M., Straube, S., Seeland, A., Kim, S.-K., Kirchner, E.A.: Measuring the improvement of the interaction comfort of a wearable exoskeleton. Int. J. Soc. Robotics **4**(3), 285–302 (2012)
4. George, L., Lécuyer, A.: An overview of research on "passive" brain-computer interfaces for implicit human-computer interaction. In: International Conference on Applied Bionics and Biomechanics ICABB 2010 - Workshop W1 "Brain-Computer Interfacing and Virtual Reality". Venice, Italy (2010)
5. Guger, C., Harkam, W., Hertnaes, C., Pfurtscheller, G.: Prosthetic control by an EEG-based brain-computer interface (BCI). In: 5th European AAATE Conference (1999)
6. Haufe, S., Treder, M.S., Gugler, M.F., Sagebaum, M., Curio, G., Blankertz, B.: EEG potentials predict upcoming emergency brakings during simulated driving. J. Neural Eng. **8**(5), 066003 (2011)
7. Iturrate, I., Montesano, L., Minguez, J.: task-dependent signal variations in EEG error-related potentials for brain-computer interfaces. J. Neural Eng. **10**, 026024 (2013)
8. Kim, S.K., Kirchner, E.A.: Classifier transferability in the detection of error related potentials from observation to interaction. In: Proceedings of the IEEE International Conference on Systems, Man, and Cybernetics, SMC 2013, Manchester, UK, 13–16 October 2013 (2013)
9. Kirchner, E.A., Metzen, J.H., Duchrow, T., Kim, S.K., Kirchner, F.: Assisting tele-manipulation operators via real-time brain reading. In: Lohweg, V., Niggemann, O. (eds.) Proceedings of Machine Learning in Real-time Application Workshop 2009. Lemgoer Schriftenreihe zur industriellen Informationstechnik, Paderborn, Germany (2009)
10. Kirchner, E.A., Wöhrle, H., Bergatt, C., Kim, S.K., Metzen, J.H., Feess, D., Kirchner, F.: Towards operator monitoring via brain reading - an EEG-based approach for space applications. In: Proceedings of 10th International Symposium on Artificial Intelligence, Robotics and Automation in Space, Sapporo (2010)
11. Kirchner, E.A., Drechsler, R.: A Formal Model for Embedded Brain Reading, vol. 40. Emerald Group Publishing Limited, Bingley (2013)
12. Kirchner, E.A., Kim, S.K.: EEG in dual-task human-machine interaction: target recognition and prospective memory. In: Proceedings of the 18th Annual Meeting of the Organization for Human Brain Mapping (2012)
13. Kirchner, E.A., Kim, S.K., Straube, S., Seeland, A., Wöhrle, H., Krell, M.M., Tabie, M., Fahle, M.: On the applicability of brain reading for predictive human-machine interfaces in robotics. PLoS ONE **8**, e81732 (2013)
14. Krell, M.M., Straube, S., Seeland, A., Wöhrle, H., Teiwes, J., Metzen, J.H., Kirchner, E.A., Kirchner, F.: pySPACE (2013). https://github.com/pyspace
15. Krell, M.M., Straube, S., Seeland, A., Wöhrle, H., Teiwes, J., Metzen, J.H., Kirchner, E.A., Kirchner, F.: pySPACE - a signal processing and classification environment in Python. Front. Neuroinf. **7**(40) (2013)

16. Kutas, M., McCarthy, G., Donchin, E.: Augmenting mental chronometry: the P300 as a measure of stimulus evaluation time. Science **197**(4305), 792–795 (1977)
17. Nijholt, A., Tan, D., Allison, B.Z., Del R Milan, J., Graimann, B.: Brain-Computer Interfaces for HCI and Games. ACM (2008)
18. Pan, S.J., Yang, Q.: A survey on transfer learning. IEEE Trans. Knowl. Data Eng. **22**(10), 1345–1359 (2010)
19. Polich, J.: Updating P300: an integrative theory of P3a and P3b. Clin. Neurophysiol. **118**(10), 2128–2148 (2007)
20. Reuderink, B.: Games and Brain-Computer Interfaces: The State of the Art. WP2 BrainGain Deliverable HMI University of Twente September 2008 (2008)
21. Rivet, B., Souloumiac, A., Attina, V., Gibert, G.: xDAWN algorithm to enhance evoked potentials: application to brain-computer interface. IEEE Trans. Biomed. Eng. **56**(8), 2035–2043 (2009)
22. Salisbury, D.F., Rutherford, B., Shenton, M.E., McCarley, R.W.: Button-pressing affects P300 amplitude and scalp topography. Clin. Neurophysiol. **112**(9), 1676–1684 (2001)
23. Seeland, A., Wöhrle, H., Straube, S., Kirchner, E.A.: Online movement prediction in a robotic application scenario. In: 2013 6th International IEEE/EMBS Conference on Neural Engineering (NER) (2013)
24. Straube, S., Krell, M.M.: How to evaluate an agent's behaviour to infrequent events? – Reliable performance estimation insensitive to class distribution. Front. Comput. Neurosci. **8**(43) (2014)
25. Wolpaw, J.R., Birbaumer, N., McFarland, D.J., Pfurtscheller, G., Vaughan, T.M.: Brain-computer interfaces for communication and control. Clin. Neurophysiol. **113**(6), 767–791 (2002)
26. Zander, T.O., Kothe, C., Jatzev, S., Gaertner, M.: Enhancing human-computer interaction with input from active and passive brain-computer interfaces. Brain-Computer Interfaces (2010)

Impact on Biker Effort of Electric Bicycle Utilization: Results from On-Road Monitoring in Lisbon, Portugal

Gonçalo Duarte$^{(\boxtimes)}$, Magno Mendes, and Patrícia Baptista

IDMEC - Instituto Superior Técnico, Universidade de Lisboa,
Av. Rovisco Pais, 1, 1049-001 Lisbon, Portugal
goncalo.duarte@tecnico.ulisboa.pt

Abstract. The objective of this work was to estimate the biker real physiological impacts (more specifically heart rate) of using electric bicycles (EB) instead of conventional bicycles (CB), by developing an appropriate methodology for on-road bio-signals data analysis. From the on-road monitoring data of 6 bikers, 2 routes and 3 bicycles in Lisbon, the results indicate a 57 % average reduction in HR variation from the use of EB, since under high power demanding situations, the electric motor attenuates human effort. The energy expenditure evaluation indicates that the total energy spent reaches ≈70 Wh/km for CB, while for EB that value is of ≈51 Wh/km of human energy (28 % lower than the CB) and ≈9 Wh/km of electricity consumption, resulting in a total of ≈60 Wh/km. As a result, using the EB allow a 14 % reduction in the total energy per km compared to the CB.

Keywords: Conventional and electric bicycles · On-road monitoring · Physiological signals · Bicycle specific power

1 Introduction

The transportation sector faces increasingly stricter energy consumption and emissions standards and accounts for 33 % of the final energy consumption, with the road transportation sector being responsible in 2011 for 82 % of that energy consumption [1].

A possibility to reduce the impact of the transportation sector, particularly in urban environments, is to decrease the demand for energy intensive modes of transportation and by promoting alternatives that provide a cheaper, less noisy and more sustainable alternative than a day-to-day car commute. Usually, some of the alternative transportation models considered are: public transportation systems (bus, trains, subway systems and others), vehicle sharing schemes (such as cars or bicycles), and alternative transportation modes such as walking, private bicycles or others [2]. From these different alternatives, the use of bicycles seems one of the more advantageous since it allows the users to move at significant speeds for short distances (typical in urban environments), with no emissions and having health benefits [3].

The use of bicycles enables people to travel longer, faster and with lower effort compared to walking, while having a low impact on environment, thus making it an

© Springer-Verlag Berlin Heidelberg 2014
H.P. da Silva et al. (Eds.): PhyCS 2014, LNCS 8908, pp. 119–133, 2014.
DOI: 10.1007/978-3-662-45686-6_8

efficient transportation mode for urban mobility. Consequently, the importance of cycling has been increasing worldwide [4, 5]. In many developing countries, namely in Asia, two-wheelers are a first affordable option towards individual mobility. In European and American cities, the deployment of city bike lane infrastructure has also been increasing, with bike sharing systems deployed having on average 200 km of bike lanes [6].

Moreover, a growing number of cities have been trying to integrate bicycles in the daily mobility of their citizens, which for some countries has resulted in a significant share of trips done using bicycles, such as the Netherlands (26 %), Denmark (18 %) and Germany (10 %) [7]. In Amsterdam for example, 38 % of all trips in 2008 were made using a bicycle, with 50 % of Amsterdam's residents riding a bike daily and 85 % riding it at least once a week [8].

While the use of conventional bicycles in an urban context has been promoted with significant success in several cities, namely Paris and London with 25000 and 8000 deployed bicycles respectively [9–11], they still have several disadvantages that hamper their widespread use. Some of the main issues identified by people when using conventional bicycles include the difficulty to travel very long distances and over hills, the possibility of arriving at a destination, such as work, sweaty or tired [12], being exposed to extreme cold or hot climates, among others. Even some cities with difficult topographies, such as Lisbon, have begun promoting the use of bicycles through the deployment of bike lanes and evaluating the possibility of having bike sharing schemes [13, 14].

Some of these issues can be resolved through the use of electric bicycles [12], which can help to reduce the effort required for performing trips as well as to reduce travel time, though at a higher cost due to the electric system and the energy used.

One of the main current applications of electric bicycles is in bike sharing systems, with several systems being deployed worldwide. The Callabike system in Aachen, Germany, has a fully electric bike sharing system with 15 electric bicycles [15]. The city of Kitakyushu in Japan also presents a full electric system with 116 bikes [16]. Cities such as St. Etienne and Poitiers in France present mixed conventional and electric bike sharing systems with a 15 % and 26 % ratio between electric and conventional bicycles respectively [17, 18].

Both conventional and electric bicycles are starting to be seen as a real option under urban environments, but the real impacts on human efforts have not yet been accounted under real operation. Also, despite the high expectations for electric bicycles, very few studies have tried to understand the real world benefits of such bicycles in an urban environment.

Regarding environmental impacts, for instance, in China the estimation of environmental impacts comparing electric bicycles with other means of transport (bus) [19] remarks that electric bikes, in a life cycle perspective which includes the well-to-tank stage, have higher emissions of SO_2 (due to burning coal for electricity production) compared to a bus. However, the emissions of other pollutants are lower in electric bike. As result, pollutant emissions are strongly related to the energy mix. The emissions associated with the production process of batteries, recycling and "dump" are also a concern.

Considering the adoption of electric bicycles, the benefits of using electrical technologies are not unanimous [20]. The potential environmental impacts, interference with traffic and safety issues, as well as the potential conflict between users of electric bikes and conventional is a concern, since the speed differences during cycling can be a problem [12].

Hence, in terms of conventional and electric bicycle usage comparison [21], a 16 % increase in average speed was verified in electric bicycle over that achieved with the conventional bicycle. Different usage strategies of the bicycle were also identified: the first strategy of using the electric bike is to use a high level of electric assist on positive slopes (uphill conditions), lowering the electric assistance levels for neutral and negative slopes; in the second strategy, the rider uses more electric assist on the positive slopes, assistance decreases in negative slopes, and reaching the lowest values in the plain areas; and the third strategy is to always use a high level of service regardless of the slope.

The biker driving dynamics represented by the speed and acceleration, combined with road topography, reflects in a power demand that must be overcome either by the biker (in a CB) or by the biker and/or the electric motor (in an EB). The quantification of human effort during cycling can be addressed [22], using an equation that includes variables such as speed, acceleration, mechanical efficiency of the bicycle, among others. Parkin states that road slope influences the energy spent by the cyclist, as well as the number of stops. In more detail, just stopping at an intersection can lead to an increase of 10 % in energy consumption.

Another issue is the quantification of effort or energy that the rider expends to complete a specific route. More importantly, whether an electric bicycle will actually decrease the effort or energy expended by the rider when compared with a conventional bicycle is also a question. There is little work developed in this field and it does not reflect real world use of conventional and electric bicycles. Therefore, a method to estimate human energy expenditure (EE) must be addressed. This method must include physiological data that can be related with energy expenditure and an analysis that could use on-road, real-world operation of electric and conventional bicycles.

A strategy for quantifying the human effort is the comparison between ventilation and heart rate as an indicator of oxygen consumption during exercise with different intensities [23]. By monitoring individuals performing different tasks (such as walking, walking carrying a certain load and intermittent work), Gastinger concluded that the most appropriate methodology is the heart rate to determine the oxygen consumption. Another possibility is a calorimeter indirect way versus heart rate monitoring to evaluate energy consumption [24]. The authors state that for determining energy consumption, in tasks of day-to-day, the two methods have very similar values, 8.6 kcal/day. However, the authors argue that the method of using the heart rate, to determine the energy consumed in the daily tasks, still needs improvements.

Accurate estimate of energy consumption through the heart rate without individual calibration laboratory can be performed [25]. The authors argue that the methodology RR_{IEST} where individual calibration of heart rate is not necessary provides an accurate and practical way to estimate the power consumption.

The comparison of two techniques to estimate the energy consumed, obtained by monitoring the heart rate, and obtained by a portable electromagnetic coil [26] allows concluding that the determination of the energy consumed using electromagnetic coil portable system is more accurate than using only the heart rate. The authors also report that would be interesting to use together, heart rate and ventilation on the determination of the energy consumed.

Several other techniques to determine the energy consumed are available or being developed, with particular reference to Doubly Labelled Water (DLW) [27]. The methods used to determine the power consumption depends on factors such as the number of individuals monitored and the monitoring period. The authors suggest that studies with few participants and short analysis periods should use the method of indirect calorimeter to obtain best results. However, for longer periods, around 3 to 4 days, it is preferable to use the method of DLW.

Although there are several techniques available, the prediction of the energy consumed during submaximal exercises could be done using heart rate readings [28]. Through tests conducted at 115 individuals in ergonomic bikes and treadmills race, the authors established an equation to determine the energy consumed by an individual during exercise. This equation includes the following variables: heart rate, age, sex and weight. The authors claim that it is possible to determine with good precision, the energy consumed using only heart rate, age, sex and weight, and without the need for individual calibration.

As can be seen, most of the techniques to estimate human energy expenditure are performed under controlled conditions – unlike the study presented, that include signals such as heart rate that can be collected while the bicycles are used.

In this sense, the objective of this work was to develop a methodology based on physiological data collection under regular bicycle operation. In more detail, this methodology allows to evaluate the use of conventional and electric bicycles for urban mobility focusing on typical hilly routes of Lisbon, quantifying their correspondent effect on human energy expenditure.

2 Methodology

2.1 On-Road Monitoring

The evaluation of electric and conventional bicycles was done through the monitoring of trips performed by 6 male different bikers (within the same age range and physical characteristics), with each biker travelling the same urban tour with both bicycles. The bikers used the electric bicycle first and the conventional bicycle after, with a minimum resting period of 1 h in-between.

The bicycles used by all bikers were the same, in order to enable a fairer evaluation, although two models of electric bicycles were evaluated. The specifications of the three bicycles used are the following:

- Conventional bicycle (CB) (Orbita Aluminio): weight of 15 kg, 21 gears;
- Electric bicycle (EB1) (QWIC Trend2): power assist electric bicycle with six levels of assistance, 25.7 kg, 7 mechanical gears and a detachable Li-ion battery with a 360 Wh capacity, provided by Prio.Energy [29]; and
- Electric bicycle (EB2) (Ekoway L1): power assist/power on demand electric bicycle with 23 kg, 6 mechanical gears and a detachable Li-ion battery with a 360 Wh capacity, provided by EcoCritério [30].

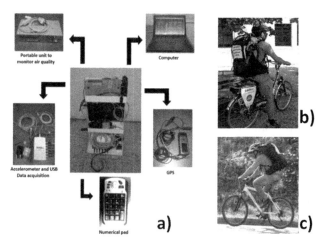

Fig. 1. MoveLab components and experimental apparatus used for the real time monitoring (a), electric bicycle (b) and conventional bicycle (c)

Each trip was monitored during the ride using a monitoring laboratory designed to assess energy and environmental impacts associated to transportation modes [21, 32]. This laboratory corresponds to a backpack weighting 12 kg that the user (pedestrian or biker) carries, as shown in Fig. 1.

This backpack is equipped with a GPS to record the dynamic profile of the trip (including location, altitude and speed), voltage and current probes to assess the levels of electric assistance, and biometric sensors (recording heart rate and breathing intensity). All these equipments were carried by the rider in the backpack. When asked to carry the backpack, the bikers saw no inconvenience since in their daily routines they already carry backpacks weighting around 5 to 8 kg.

All the equipment is connected to a laptop running a purposely developed software in LabView to synchronize and record the data at 1 Hz, throughout the trip. The technical description of the equipment used is presented in Table 1.

Additionally, bioPLUX Research hardware and software acquiring physiological data were used simultaneously. In order to synchronize the two sources of data (LabView and bioPLUX Research), a force sensor was adapted to the numeric pad.

Table 1. Technical description of the equipment used in MoveLab

Monitoring equipment	Data acquired	Temporal resolution of data (Hz)
GPS (Garmin GPS map 76CSx)	Speed (km/h), altitude (m), location	1
Voltage and current probes (Fluke i1010)	Voltage, current	1
bioPLUX Research	Heart rate, Breathing rate	200

This way, when the biker pressed Enter, this signal was recorded either in LabView and in the Plux software. Since the bio-signals require a high frequency data logging, a minimum of 200 samples per second were collected while the biker was riding. Due to the different temporal resolution physiologic data was post processed into a second by second time basis.

2.2   Data Collection and Processing

The GPS collects speed, location and also altitude information via an integrated barometric altimeter. The altimeter was adequately installed inside the backpack, avoiding pressure fluctuations due to movement that could affect the readings and an external antenna was used to avoid GPS signal losses.

Voltage probes were installed directly in the bicycle battery terminals, while current measurements were done on the circuit that connects the battery to the electric motor. The signals provided by the probes were collected by a National Instruments DAQ board installed also on the backpack. For battery voltage signal a voltage divider circuit was placed before the DAQ board to account for the 0–10 V limit of the acquisition device.

Both GPS and battery data were collected in a PC using a program developed in LabView by the authors to integrate the different communication protocols (serial port and NMEA protocol for GPS and analog data via USB port for the voltage and current collected in the DAQ board) that allows to synchronize the data, capturing all the equipment readings in a 1 Hz basis. A solid-state disk PC was used to avoid data loss while in motion.

The bioPLUX Research tool was used to collect heart rate and breathing rate. This information was collected at 200 Hz using PLUX software. Post processing of data included the conversion of the data to 1 Hz basis. It should be noticed that breathing rate measured is very sensible to vibration under regular bicycle operation, therefore it was decided not to use this data.

GPS readings of speed were used to post process distance travelled, acceleration and road grade. Altitude and distance were used to determine the trip road grade using an algorithm that, for each point of the trip, finds the points 50 m before and after and uses this information to establish a second order polynomial fit based on three points of distance and altitude. The derivative of the polynomial fit in the studied point allows determining road grade, which is presented in rad.

Battery data was used to determine, at each point of the trip, the power provided by battery to the electric motor, according to the biker demands, and integrate this data along the trip to find the cumulative energy spent on the predefined tour.

The collected data allows to understand and quantify how riders changed their use profile (in terms of speed and acceleration), changing from a conventional bicycle to an electric one. Similarly, the physiological impacts on the adoption of an electric bicycle versus the conventional were addressed using the physiological data, with the final goal of providing an estimate of the human energy expenditure.

2.3   Monitored Tours

To compare the use of conventional and electric bicycles, round-trip tours of approximately 8.5 km and 5.7 km were performed by each biker, in Lisbon, with both bicycles. One of the tours consisted on going from Instituto Superior Técnico (IST) main campus to downtown Lisbon and back, passing through the top of the Parque Eduardo VII and Avenida da Liberdade on both ways. With this tour, the bikers crossed different parts of the city of Lisbon including traffic intensive avenues, side roads with very little traffic and a street with a bike lane. The other tour was carried in the EXPO 98 area, simulating a journey in a leisure place with low traffic conditions. In terms of topography, the tours had significant slopes, as summarized in Table 2.

Table 2. Selected tours

Route	Distance (km)	Average positive slope (rad)	Average negative slope (rad)
R1	8.54	0.037	−0.029
R2	5.66	0.020	−0.017

2.4   Methodology for Data Analysis

The analysis used in this work is based on Vehicle Specific Power (VSP) to estimate the power demand by vehicles, which combines speed (v), acceleration (a) and road grade (θ). This methodology allows comparing different technologies under similar power requirements. It is traditionally used on light-duty vehicles [31] and its generic definition, which includes the forces applied to a moving body, is presented in Eq. 1. The coefficients of the equation are adjusted according to the typology of vehicle monitored [32].

$$VSP = \frac{\frac{d}{dt}\left(E_{Kinetic} + E_{Potential}\right) + F_{Rolling} \cdot v + F_{Aerodynamic} \cdot v}{m}$$

$$= v \cdot \left[a \cdot (1 + \varepsilon_i) + g \cdot sen(\theta) + g \cdot C_R\right] + \frac{1}{2} \cdot \rho_a \cdot C_D \cdot \frac{A}{m} \cdot v^3 \qquad (1)$$

Table 3. Coefficient values for the variables included in BSP

Variables	Values
ε	0.01
g (m/s^2)	9.81
C_R	0.008
C_D	1.2
A (m^2)	0.5
$m_{bicycle}$ (kg)	18
m_{biker} (kg)	70
ρ_a (kg/m^3)	1.2

For the specific case of bicycles, the values used for the coefficients were select to best fit the typical bicycles uses in daily commuting, according with Wilson [33], resulting in the Bicycle Specific Power methodology (BSP). In order to include both conventional and electric bicycles in the BSP methodology, a bicycle weight that already account for the increasing mass of electric solutions was selected. The remaining properties are similar for conventional and electric bicycles, as presented in Table 3.

In this case, the coefficients used, adapted to typical utility bicycles based on literature values [33], allow to obtain the bicycle specific power (BSP), in W/kg, as defined by Eq. 2:

$$BSP = v \cdot [1.01 \cdot a + 9.81 \cdot sen(\theta) + 0.078] + 0.0041 \cdot v^3 \qquad (2)$$

Correspondingly to the VSP methodology, the BSP is also divided in modes that cover the full spectrum of the bicycle operation, according to the following formulation: group points with similar BSP values (in W/kg); each BSP mode must include more than 1 % of the total trip time, providing representativeness for each mode; and the number of modes is such that the total trip time is not concentrated in a limited number of points. Table 4 presents the modes (or bins) used in this work and the respective range of power per mass.

Table 4. Binning method for BSP

BSP mode	Definition	BSP mode	Definition	BSP mode	Definition
<-4	BSP < -1	-1	-1 ≤ BSP < 0	3	2 ≤ BSP < 3
-4	-4 ≤ BSP < -3	0	BSP = 0	4	3 ≤ BSP < 4
-3	-3 ≤ BSP < -2	1	0 ≤ BSP < 1	>4	BSP > 4
-2	-2 ≤ BSP < -1	2	1 ≤ BSP < 2		

The percentage of time spent in each BSP mode for the conventional and electric bicycles is presented in Fig. 2(a, b). For negative modes, the driving profile is very similar for both bicycles. Conversely, on positive BSP modes, the electric bicycle present a higher share of time spent in high BSP modes (higher power demands). This is due to the electric assistance, which allows traveling at high speeds on higher slopes and combinations of higher speeds and acceleration, etc.

Figure 3 presents the energy rate spent at each BSP mode, on average, for the electric bicycles studied, using the 1 Hz data from voltage and current provided by the battery, measured under on-road conditions. As expected, the energy rate increases with BSP mode, showing the dominance of electric assist on these modes.

Although the data presented so far allows taking conclusions about usage patterns of biker in EB and CB, in both electric and conventional bicycles it is necessary to determine the physiological impacts of each technology and the respective human energy expenditure to address the total energy impacts.

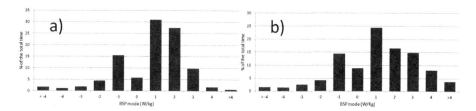

Fig. 2. Time distribution (%) per BSP mode for: (a) conventional bicycle; (b) two electric bicycles.

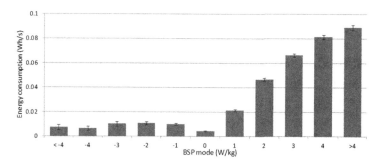

Fig. 3. Electricity consumption for the electric bicycles as a function of BSP.

3   Results

The main goal was to relate trip dynamic variables (expressed by BSP) with HR variations. Hence, since BSP aggregates trip information of speed, acceleration and slope, its influence on heart rate was analyzed. Additionally, since HR differ from person to person, this evaluation was performed using its derivate, $\left(\frac{\Delta HR}{\Delta t}\right)$, and not its absolute value. Furthermore, since HR is an indirect unit of energy, $\left(\frac{\Delta HR}{\Delta t}\right)$ expresses the variation of Energy in a period of time, hence a measure of Power.

Due to the existence of some noise in the HR signal due to movement and vibration, the HR and BSP second by second data was aggregated in a minute by minute basis. In total, over 8 h of data was collected.

Figure 4 presents a clear relation between BSP and $\left(\frac{\Delta HR}{\Delta t}\right)$. For mode 0, that corresponds to the biker stopped, a reduction in $\left(\frac{\Delta HR}{\Delta t}\right)$ is observed, which means that the biker reduced his HR in this condition, compared with the previous riding condition (thus $\left(\frac{\Delta HR}{\Delta t}\right) < 0$). For positive BSP modes, which require more power from the biker, positive variations in HR are observed due to the increased human effort. As a result, for increasing BSP modes, increasing positive variation in $\left(\frac{\Delta HR}{\Delta t}\right)$ are observed. BSP mode > 4 has few riding data points, which justifies its divergence. For negative BSP modes, which usually correspond to braking or descent situation, reductions in HR/s are observed.

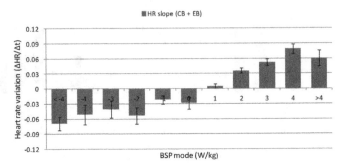

Fig. 4. Influence of BSP in (ΔHR/Δt) for the total data collected.

The collected data was also disaggregated according to conventional and electric bicycle. Figure 5 presents the $\left(\frac{\Delta HR}{\Delta t}\right)$ average results according to the usage of conventional or electric bicycle. Over 4 h of data are represented both for electric and conventional bicycles (considering the average of two electric and conventional bicycles that were monitored). The variations in HR/s are lower for the electric bicycle. That is mainly visible in positive BSP modes, where higher power demand is observed. For the electric bicycle, having the electric motor assistance, helps reducing the human effort and, consequently, variations in HR/s are lower. For negative BSP modes, that difference is not so visible, with both bicycles leading to reductions in HR. It should be noticed that for the highest BSP mode, the trend is not followed due to the lack of points to fully characterize those conditions.

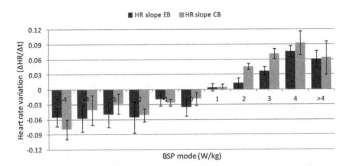

Fig. 5. Influence of BSP in (ΔHR/Δt) for conventional (gray) and electric bicycles (black).

In order to obtain an average HR variation at the end of the trip, the temporal distribution of BSP was multiplied by the HR variations. Table 5 presents the average $\sum(\Delta HR)$ for each type of bicycle. The electric bicycle leads to lower values compared to the conventional one, with an average 57 % reduction.

The next step was to analyze the human energy expenditure (EE) associated to each trip. This corresponds to the energy spent by the biker to drive the bicycle. According to the literature review [26–28] this corresponds to an accurate approximation to

Table 5. Results of $\sum(\Delta HR)$ for CB and EB.

Bicycle	$\sum(\Delta HR)$
EB	0.59
CB	1.37

Table 6. Quantification of Energy Expenditure (EE) from Heart Rate (HR).

Source	EE
[28]	EE = gender $\times$ $(-55.0969 + 0.6309 \times HR + 0.1988 \times weight + 0.2017 \times age) + (1 - gender) \times (-20.4022 + 0.4472 \times HR - 0.1263 \times weight + 0.074 \times age)$ EE in kJ/min; HR in BPM; gender = 1 for man and 2 for woman. In this study, all biker were male, with an average age of 28 and average weight of 70 kg
[26]	EE = $0.103 \times HR - 4.795$ EE in kcal/min; HR in BPM
[27]	EE = $0.0056 \times HR^2 - 0.6908 \times HR + 26.532$ EE in kJ/min; HR in BPM
Average equation	$\mathbf{EE = (9 \times 10^{-6}) \times HR^2 + 0.0006 \times HR - 0.0449}$

account with the energy the body requires during physical activity. The estimation of EE can be performed using the equations presented in Table 6.

The 3 equations presented can be represented simultaneously to obtain Fig. 6 and an average equation was obtained (Table 6) that was used for the purpose of this study.

Using the 8 h of physiologic data (divided in 4 h for CB and the remaining for EB) and recurring to the obtained average equation (Table 6), the EE value was estimated to each second of the trip. The next logical step was to group points with similar BSP conditions, to obtain a representative EE value associated to each BSP mode. This data is presented in Fig. 7, with the gray bars representing CB and the black bars representing the EB.

Figure 7 presents the results of multiplying the EE profiles (in Wh/s) by each trip BSP time distribution, for EB and CB. This way, the EE (in Wh) for each BSP mode is

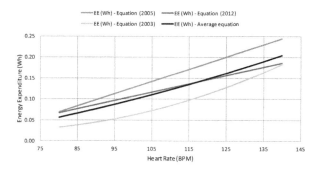

Fig. 6. Energy Expenditure as a function of Heart Rate.

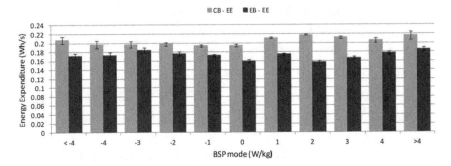

Fig. 7. Energy Expenditure for each BSP mode for CB and EB.

obtained. Adding the EE at each BSP mode and dividing by the trip distance, an estimate of the human energy expenditure per kilometer (Wh/km) is assigned for each trip and technology used (conventional or electric).

In order to obtain the total energy consumption (human and electric), an approach similar to the one described previously was used for estimating electric use, according to the consumption profile distribution from Fig. 3, instead of Fig. 7.

Figure 8 presents an estimate of the total energy per kilometer (human plus electric in electric bicycle and human only in conventional bicycle). For the conventional bicycle the total energy is around 69.8 Wh/km, while the electric bicycle presents 50.6 Wh/km of human energy (less 27.5 % compared with conventional bicycle) and 9.2 Wh/km of electric consumption, resulting in a total of 59.8 Wh/km. Therefore, the total energy per kilometer is 14.3 % lower in the electric bicycle than in the conventional. It is worth mentioning, that the life cycle energy impacts could also include the food requirement of the bikers to move both bicycles. However, for simplification reasons this layer was assumed to be comparable.

With the data collected, it was not possible to effectively estimate the efficiency of the electric motor and the human body while cycling. However, it is possible to obtain a set of acceptable values for those efficiencies. Therefore, it was assumed that to travel the distance of one kilometer it is necessary the same energy, independently of using the electric and conventional bicycle (Eq. 3).

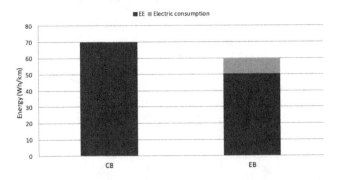

Fig. 8. Total energy expenditure for CB and EB.

$$E_{req\_CB} = (\varepsilon_H \times EE_{CB}) \Leftrightarrow E_{req\_EB} = (\varepsilon_H \times EE_{EB})$$
$$+ (\varepsilon_M \times \text{Electricity consumption}) \Leftrightarrow E_{req\_CB} = E_{req\_EB} \quad (3)$$

Where E_{req_CB} is the required energy for CB; E_{req_EB} is the required energy for EB; ε_H – is the human body efficiency; ε_M is electric motor efficiency; EE_{CB} is the EE for CB; and EE_{EB} is the EE for EB. Using to Eq 3 and assuming a range of typical efficiency values for an electric motor, between 60 to 95 %, the range of human efficiency can be estimated, as presented in Fig. 9. As a result, while cycling, the efficiency of human body, theoretically, ranges from 30 % to 45 %.

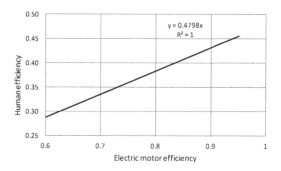

Fig. 9. Human efficiency versus electric motor efficiency.

4   Conclusions

This research work addressed the use of conventional and electric bicycles in real world conditions, in order to estimate its impacts on physiological signals, in more detail, in heart rate and human energy expenditure. For this purpose, a methodology to quantify the power required to overcome a drive cycle was adapted from vehicle to bicycles, resulting in the BSP methodology. The application of this methodology used as basis data from the monitoring of 6 bikers using both CB and EB, over 114 km in the city of Lisbon, Portugal, showing that EB allow reaching higher BSP modes. However, the developed methodology is not city or route specific and can be applied elsewhere.

The impact on heart rate from shifting from conventional bicycle usage to electric bicycle usage was estimated. An average 57 % reduction in HR variations was found for the use of EB in typical trips since, in high BSP modes that represent power demanding situation, the electric motor comes in action, avoiding human effort.

Moreover, a methodology was established to quantify the energy expenditure, based on heart rate data measured under regular bicycle operation, associated to the human effort that results from using the bicycles. For the conventional bicycle the total human energy expenditure reaches ≈70 Wh/km, while the electric bicycle presents ≈51 Wh/km of human energy (27.5 % lower than the conventional bicycle) and ≈9 Wh/km of electric consumption, resulting in a total of ≈60 Wh/km. Consequently, the total energy per kilometer is 14.3 % lower in the electric bicycle compared to the conventional.

In all, an innovative method of quantifying the benefits for the biker of using electric bicycles was developed, resulting in significant reduction in heart rate variations, as well as, considerable energy efficiency improvements. Using all the modal information from Figs. 4 and 8 regarding electric and human energy rates, combined with BSP modal distribution for any route (as is presented in Figs. 2 and 3), this methodology allows estimating the total energy expenditure (human and electric), electric autonomy, as well as HR variations, according to the trip profile. As a result, this methodology can be applied to evaluate the potential use of EB in specific situation, namely bike-sharing routes, providing significant support to bike-sharing systems design and deployment.

Future work will be performed to include other physiological signals (such as breathing rate or ventilation rate) to obtain a more accurate estimation of the human power.

Acknowledgements. The authors would like to acknowledge the sponsors of the research: Prio.e and Eco-critério. Thanks are also due to Fundação para a Ciência e Tecnologia for the Post-Doctoral financial support (SFRH /BPD /79684 /2011).

References

1. EUROSTAT: Environment and Energy, EUROPA Eurostat – Data Navigation Tree, http://ec.europa.eu/eurostat (2013) [cited May 2013]
2. Wang, R.: Autos, transit and bicycles: Comparing the costs in large Chinese cities. Transp. Policy **18**, 139–146 (2011)
3. Lindsay, G., Macmillan, A., Woodward, A.: Moving urban trips from cars to bicycles: impact on health and emissions. Aus. New Zealand J. Public Health **35**(1), 54–60 (2011)
4. Urban Audit: Urban Audit: Welcome to the Urban Audit web site. http://www.urbanaudit.org/. [cited October 2012]
5. Freemark, Y.: Transit mode share trends looking steady; Rail appears to encourage non-automobile commutes, The Transport Politic (2010). http://www.thetransportpolitic.com/2010/10/13/transit-mode-share-trends-looking-steady-rail-appears-to-encourage-non-automobile-commutes/. (Cited October 2012)
6. Baptista, P.: On-road monitoring of electric bicycles and its use in bike-sharing systems. In: Silva, C. (ed.) Grid Electrified Vehicles: Performance, Design and Environmental Impacts. Nova Science Publishers Inc, New York (2013)
7. Buehler, R., Pucher, J.: Walking and Cycling in Western Europe and the United States - Trends, Policies, and Lessons. TR News May–June 2012: Active Transportation: Implementing the Benefits (2012)
8. Gardner, G.: Power to the pedals. World Watch Mag. **23**(4) (2010). http://www.worldwatch.org/node/6456
9. Vélib: Vélib - Bikesharing scheme in Paris (2012). http://en.velib.paris.fr/. (Cited October 2012)
10. Barclays Cycle Hire: Barclays Cycle Hire - Bikesharing in London (2012). http://www.tfl.gov.uk/roadusers/cycling/14808.aspx. (Cited October 2012)
11. Lathia, N., Ahmed, S., Capra, L.: Measuring the impact of opening the London shared bicycle scheme to casual users. Transp. Res. Part C Emer. Technol. **22**, 88–102 (2012)

12. Dill, J., Rose, G.: E-bikes and transportation policy: Insights from early adopters. In: 91th Annual Meeting of the Transportation Research Board (2012)
13. Galp Energia: Ciclovias e percursos pedonais (2012). http://www.galpenergia.com/PT/sustentabilidade/eficiencia-energetica/na-sociedade/o-desafio-da-mobilidade-sustentavel/Paginas/Ciclovias-e-percursos-pedonais.aspx. (Cited September 2012)
14. Martinez, L., Caetano, L., Eiró, T., Cruz, F.: An optimisation algorithm to establish the location of stations of a mixed fleet biking system: An application to the city of Lisbon. In: 15th Edition of the Euro Working Group on Transportation, Paris (2012)
15. Callabike: Callabike bike sharing system (2012). http://www.callabike-interaktiv.de/. (Cited October 2012)
16. The Bike-sharing Blog: Japanese Bike-share is Electric (2011). http://bike-sharing.blogspot.pt/2011/06/japanese-bike-share-is-electric.html. (Cited October 2012)
17. VéliVert: VéliVert - Bikesharing scheme in Saint-Etienne (2012). http://www.velivert.fr/. (Cited October 2012)
18. Cap'Vélo: Se déplacer à vélo en Grand Poitiers - Bikesharing scheme in Saint-Etienne (2012). http://www.grandpoitiers.fr/c__54_163__Louer_un_velo.html. (Cited October 2012)
19. Cherry, C., Weinert, J., Xinmiao, Y.: Comparative environmental impacts of electric bikes in China. Transp. Res. Part D **14**, 281–290 (2009)
20. Cherry, C.: and R. Cervero, Use characteristics and mode choice behavior of electric bike users in China, Transport Policy **14**, 247–257 (2007)
21. Baptista, P., et al.: On road evaluation of electric and conventional bicycles for urban mobility (submitted to Transport Policy) (2013)
22. Parkin, J.: The importance of human effort in planning networks. In: NECTAR Workshop Abstract (2011)
23. Gastinger, S., et al.: A comparison between ventilation and heart rate as indicator of oxygen uptake during different intensities of exercise. J. Sports Sci. Med. **9**, 110–118 (2010)
24. Yu, Z., et al.: Comparison of heart rate monitoring with indirect calorimetry for energy expenditure evaluation. J. Sport Health Sci. **1**, 178–183 (2012)
25. Pulkkinen, A., Saalasti, S., Rusko, H.: Energy expenditure can be accurately estimated from HR without individual laboratory calibration. In: 52nd Annual Meeting of the American College of Sports Medicine, Nashville, Tennessee, USA (2005)
26. Gastinger, S., et al.: Energy expenditure estimate by heart-rate monitor and a portable electromagnetic-coil system. Int. J. Sport Nutr. Exerc. Metab. **22**, 117–130 (2012)
27. Ainslie, P., Reilly, T., Westerterp, K.: Estimating human energy expenditure: A review of techniques with particular reference to doubly labelled water. Sports Med. **33**, 683–698 (2003)
28. Keytel, L., et al.: Prediction of energy expenditure from heart rate monitoring during submaximal exercise. J. Sports Sci. **23**, 289–297 (2005)
29. Prio Energy: Prio Energy - Electric Mobility (2012). http://www.prioenergy.com/. Cited October 2012
30. Eco-critério (2013). http://www.ecocriterio.pt/
31. Jiménez-Palacios, J.: Understanding and Quantifying Motor Vehicle Emissions with Vehicle Specific Power and TILDAS Remote Sensing. Massachusets Institute of Technology, Cambridge (1999)
32. Baptista, P., et al.: Scenarios for electric bicycle use: From on-road monitoring to possible impacts of large introduction. In: NECTAR Conference on Dynamics of Global and Local Networks. São Miguel Island, Azores (Portugal) (2013)
33. Wilson, D.G.: Bicycling Science. The MIT Press, Cambridge (2004)

Human Factors

Learning Effective Models of Emotions from Physiological Signals: The Seven Principles

Rui Henriques[1][✉] and Ana Paiva[2]

[1] KDBIO, Inesc-ID, Instituto Superior Técnico, Universidade de Lisboa,
Lisboa, Portugal
`rmch@tecnico.ulisboa.pt`
[2] GAIPS, Inesc-ID, Instituto Superior Técnico, Universidade de Lisboa,
Lisboa, Portugal
`ana.s.paiva@tecnico.ulisboa.pt`

Abstract. Learning effective models from emotion-elicited physiological responses for the classification and description of emotions is increasingly required to derive accurate analysis from affective interactions. Despite the relevance of this task, there is still lacking an integrative view of existing contributions. Additionally, there is no agreement on how to deal with the differences of physiological responses across individuals, and on how to learn from flexible sequential behavior and subtle but meaningful spontaneous variations of the signals. In this work, we rely on empirical evidence to define *seven principles* for a robust mining physiological signals to recognize and characterize affective states. These principles compose a coherent and complete roadmap for the development of new methods for the analysis of physiological signals. In particular, these principles address the current over-emphasis on feature-based models by including critical generative views derived from different streams of research, including multivariate data analysis and temporal data mining. Additionally, we explore how to use background knowledge related with the experimental setting and psychophysiological profiles from users to shape the learning of emotion-centered models. A methodology that integrates these principles is proposed and validated using signals collected during human-to-human and human-to-robot affective interactions.

Keywords: Physiological signals · Emotion recognition · Emotion description · Affective interactions

1 Introduction

Physiological signals are increasingly monitored to measure, describe and dynamically shape affective interactions. Although many methods have been proposed for an emotion-centered analysis of physiological signals [12,31], the existing contributions have not yet been coherently integrated. Additionally, existing methods suffer from three major problems. First, there is no agreement on how to deal with individual differences and with spontaneous variations of the

© Springer-Verlag Berlin Heidelberg 2014
H.P. da Silva et al. (Eds.): PhyCS 2014, LNCS 8908, pp. 137–155, 2014.
DOI: 10.1007/978-3-662-45686-6_9

signals. Second, there is an emphasis on models learned from statistical features that are not able to consider flexible sequential behavior that is often associated with the generative modeling of physiological responses. Finally, there is a clear gap on how to use background knowledge, such as psychophysiological traits of the users and annotations related with the experimental setting, to enhance the performance of the classification models.

To address these problems, a coherent set of seven principles is proposed to guide the mining of physiological signals for an effective emotion recognition and description. These principles were synthesized from initial empirical evidence from the application of advanced techniques from machine learning and signal processing over physiological data collected during affective interactions. They provide an integrated and up-to-date view on how to disclose and characterize affective states from physiological signals. A methodology that coherently integrated these principles is, additionally, proposed.

This paper is structured as follows. Section 2 motivates the need for an integrative and extended view of existing dispersed contributions. We introduce the background to address this problem and survey relevant work. Section 3 defines the seven principles and plugs them within a coherent methodology. Section 4 provides initial empirical evidence for the utility of the seven principles using signals collected from different experimental studies. Finally, concluding remarks and major implications are provided.

2   Background

Monitoring physiological responses is increasingly necessary to derive accurate analysis from affective interactions and to dynamically respond or adapt these interactions. The use of physiological signals to measure, describe and affect human-robot interactions is critical since they track subtle but significant affective changes that are hard to perceive, and are neither prone to social masking nor have the heightened context-sensitivity of image, audio and survey-based analysis. However, their complex, variable and subjective expression within and among individuals pose key challenges for an adequate modeling of emotions.

Definition 1. *Consider a set of annotated signals $D = (x_1, .., x_m)$, where each instance is a tuple $x_i = (\vec{y}, a_1, .., a_n, c)$ where $\vec{y}$ is the signal (either univariate or multivariate), a_i is an annotation related with the subject or experimental setting, and c is the labeled emotion or stimulus. Given D, the emotion recognition task aims learn a model M to label a new unlabeled instance $(\vec{y}, a_1, .., a_n)$. Emotion description task aims to learn a model M that characterizes the major properties of $\vec{y}$ signal for each emotion c.*

The goal of emotion recognition and description is to (dynamically) access someone's feelings from (streaming) signals[1]. The multivariate signal condition in the definition allows for the combination of different physiological modalities to compose $\vec{y}$ as long as they are monitored along the same temporal window. In this case, we assume that proper dedicated pre-processing techniques are applied over each modality, such as smoothing, low-pass filtering and neutralization of cyclic behavior for respiratory and cardiac signals [17]. Emotion description as it is defined has been seen as an optional byproduct of emotion recognition from physiological signals. Previous work by the authors [9] surveys existing challenges of emotion description and extends existing supervised and unsupervised models to guarantee their utility as descriptors[2].

Emotion recognition from physiological signals has been applied in the context of human-robot interaction [14,16], human-computer interaction [26], social interaction [4], sophisticated virtual adaptive scenarios [27], among others [1,12]. Depending on the goal of the task, multiple physiological signals, categories of experiments and models of emotions can be adopted. Table 1 synthesizes the major directions of existing research according to three dimensions. Despite the large number of contributions within each of these dimensions [12,31], there are still lacking integrative principles for learning effective models of emotions from physiological signals.

A first drawback of existing emotion-centered studies is the absence of learned principles to mine the signals. Although multiple models are compared using accuracy levels, there is no in-depth analysis of the underlying behavior of these models and no guarantees regarding their statistical significance. Additionally, there is no assessment on how their performance varies for alternative experimental settings.

---

[1] Illustrative applications include: measuring human interaction with *artificial agents*, assisting *clinical research* (emotion-centered understanding of addiction, affect dysregulation, alcoholism, anxiety, autism, attention deficit, depression, drug reaction, epilepsy, menopause, locked-in syndrome, pain management, phobias and desensitization therapy, psychiatric counseling, schizophrenia, sleep disorders, and sociopathy), studying the effect of body posture and exercises in *well-being*, disclosing responses to *marketing* and suggestive interfaces, reducing *conflict* in schools and prisons through the early detection of hampering behavior, fostering *education* by relying on emotion-centered feedback to escalate behavior and increase motivation, development of (pedagogic) *games*, and *self-awareness* enhancement.

[2] Learning descriptive models of emotions from labeled signals should satisfy four major *requirements*: *flexibility* (descriptive models cope with the complex and variable physiological expression of emotions within and among individuals), *discriminative power* (descriptive models capture and enhance the different physiological responses among emotions at an individual and group level), *completeness* (descriptive models contain all of the discriminative properties and, when the reconstitution of the signal behavior is relevant, of flexible sequential abstractions), and *usability* (descriptive models are compact and the abstractions of physiological responses are easily interpretable).

Table 1. Research dimensions for recognizing and describing emotions from physiological data.

Physiological signals	Illustrating, electrodermal activity has been used to identify engagement and excitement states [11], respiratory volume and rate to recognize negative-valenced emotions, heat contractile activity to separate positive-valenced emotions [32], as well as brain and body activity (through electroencephalography and electromyography) to isolate emotional states [4]. Depending on the target emotions to assess, a combination of different modalities is often desirable [12]
Approach	The experimental setting of existing studies can be grouped according four different axes [29,30]: the properties of the selected stimuli (discrete vs. continuous), general factors related with user dependency (studies with single vs. multiple subjects), subjectivity of the stimuli (high-agreement stimuli vs. self-report emotions), and the analysis time of the signal (static vs. dynamic)
Models of emotions	The most applied models are the *discrete* model [6] centered on five-to-eight categories of emotions and the *dimensional* valence-arousal model [15] where emotions are described according to a pleasantness and intensity matrix. Other models include the Ellsworth's dimensions and agency [23], Weiner's attributions and recent work focused on recognizing states that are a complex mix of emotions ("the state of finding annoying usability problems") [25]

A second drawback is related with the fact that these studies rely on simple pre-processing techniques and feature-driven models. First, pre-processing steps are centered on the removal of contaminations and on simplistic normalization procedures. These techniques are insufficient to deal with differences on responses among subjects and with the isolation of spontaneous variations of the signal.

Second, even in the presence of expressive features, models are not able to effectively accommodate flexible sequential behavior. For instance, a rising or recovering behavior may be described by specific motifs sensitive to sub-peaks or displaying a logarithmic decaying. The weak-differentiation among responses and lack of complementary generative views leads to rigid models of emotions.

The task of this work is to identify a set of consistent principles to address these drawbacks, thus improving emotion recognition rates.

3   Solution

Relying on experimental evidence, seven principles were defined to surpass the limitations of traditional models for emotion recognition from physiological signals. The impact of adopting these principles were validated over electrodermal activity, facial expression and skin temperature signals. Nevertheless, these principles can be tested for any other physiological signal after the neutralization of cyclic behavior (e.g. respiratory and cardiac signals) and/or the application of smoothing and low-pass filters.

3.1   The Seven Principles

#1: *Use representations able to handle individual differences of responses*

Problem: The differences of physiological responses for a single emotion are often related with experimental conditions, such as the placement of sensors or unregulated environment, and with specific psychophysiological properties of the subjects, such as lability and current mood. These undesirable differences affect both the: *(i)* amplitude axis (varying baseline levels and peak-variations of responses), and the *(ii)* temporal axis (varying latency, rising and recovery time of responses).

On one hand, recognition rates degrade as a result of an increased modeling complexity due to these differences. On the other hand, when normalizing signals along the amplitude-time axes, we are discarding absolute behavior that is often critical to distinguish emotions. Additionally, common normalization procedures are not adequate since the signal baseline and response amplitude may not be correlated (e.g. high baseline does not mean heightened elicited responses).

Solution: A new representation of the signal that minimizes individual differences should be adopted, and combined with the original signal to learn the target model.

While many representations for time series exist [19], they either scale poorly as the cardinality is not changed or require previous access to all the signal preventing a dynamic analysis of the signal. Symbolic ApproXimation (SAX) satisfies these requirements and offers a lower-bounding guarantee. SAX behavior can be synthesized in two steps. First, the signal is transformed into a Piecewise Aggregate Approximated (PAA) representation. Second, the PAA signal is symbolized into a discrete string. A Gaussian distribution is used to produce symbols with equiprobability from statistical breakpoints [18]. Unlike other representations, the Gaussian distribution for amplitude control smooths the problem of subjects with baseline levels and response variations not correlated.

Amplitude differences can be corrected with respect to all stimuli, to a target stimulus, to all subjects, or to a specific subject. To treat temporal differences, two strategies can be adopted. First, signals can be used as-is (with their different numerosity) and given as input to sequential learners, which are able to deal with this aspect. Note, for instance, the robustness of hidden Markov models on detecting hand-writing text with different sizes in [2]. Second, the use of piecewise aggregation analysis, such as provided by SAX, can be used to normalize numerosity differences.

#2: *Account for relevant signal variations*

Problem: Motifs and features sensitive to sub-peaks are critical for emotion recognition (e.g. spontaneous variations of the electrodermal signal hold the potential to separate anger from fear responses [1]). However, traditional methods rely on fixed amplitude-thresholds to detect informative signal variations, which became easily corrupted due to the individual subject differences. Additionally, when cardinality is reduced, relevant sub-peaks disappear.

Solution: Two strategies can be adopted. First, a representation to enhance local variations, referred as local-angle. The signal is partitioned in thin time-partitions and the angle associated with the signal variation for each partition is computed and translated into symbols based on break-points computed from the input number of symbols. Similarly to SAX, the angle break points are also defined assuming a Gaussian distribution. Figure 1 provides the structural codification of this representation. Illustrating, when adopting a 6-dim alphabet, the following SAX-based univariate signal: <17,13,15,14,18,19,16,14,13,12,16,16>, would be translated into the following local-angle representation: <0,4,1,5,5,0,1,1,1,5,4>.

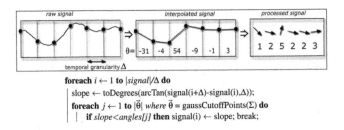

```
foreach i ← 1 to |signal|/Δ do
    slope ← toDegrees(arcTan(signal(i+Δ)-signal(i),Δ));
    foreach j ← 1 to |θ⃗| where θ⃗ = gaussCutoffPoints(Σ) do
        if slope<angles[j] then signal(i) ← slope; break;
```

Fig. 1. Pre-processing of a univariate signal using local angles with four symbols.

Second, multiple SAX representations can be adopted using different cardinalities. While mapping the raw signals into low-cardinal signals is useful to capture smoothed behavior (e.g. alphabet size less than 8), a map into high-cardinal signals is able to capture more delineated behavior (e.g. alphabet size above 10). One model can be learned for each representation, with the joint probability being computed to label a response.

#3: Include flexible sequential behavior

Problem: Although sequential learning is the natural option for audio-and-visual signals, the existing models for emotion recognition mainly rely on extracted features. Feature-extraction methods are not able to capture flexible behavior (e.g. motifs underlying complex rising and decaying responses) and are strongly dependent on directive thresholds (e.g. peak amplitude to compute frequency measures).

Solution: Generative models learned from sequential data, such as recurrent neural networks or dynamic Bayesian networks, can be adopted to satisfy this principle [2]. In particular, hidden Markov models (HMMs) are an attractive option due to their stability, simplicity and flexible parameter-control [22]. The core task is to learn the generation and transition probabilities of a hidden automaton (that follows a Markov constraint) per emotion. This is done by maximizing a likelihood function using an efficient forward-backward algorithm until convergence [2,22]. The core task is to learn the generation and transition probabilities of a hidden automaton for each emotion. Given a non-labeled signal, we can assess the probability of being generated by each learned model.

The parameterization of HMMs must be based on the signal properties (e.g. high dimensionality leads to an increased number of hidden states). Alternative architectures, such as fully-interconnected or left-to-right architectures, can be considered.

From the conducted experiments, an analysis of the learned emissions from the main path of left-to-right HMM architectures revealed emerging rising and recovering responses following sequential patterns with flexible displays (e.g. exponential and "stairs"-appearance behavior).

#4: Integrate sequential and feature-driven models

Problem: Since sequential learners capture the overall behavior of physiological responses, they are not able to highlight specific discriminative properties of the signal. Often such discriminative properties are adequately described by simple features.

Solution: Feature-driven and sequential models should be integrated as they provide different but complementary views. One option is to rely on a post-voting stage. A second option is to use one model to discriminate the less probable emotions, and to use such constraints on the remaining model.

Feature-driven models have been widely researched and are centered on four major steps: pre-processing, feature extraction, feature selection and feature-based learning [12, 17]. Table 2 surveys the contributions from different streams of research to deliver effective feature-driven models.

#5: Use subject's traits to shape the model

Problem: Subjects with different psychophysiological profiles tend to have different physiological responses for the same stimuli. Modeling responses for emotions without this prior knowledge hampers the learning task since the models have to define multiple paths or generalize responses in order to accommodate such alternative expressions of an emotion due to profile differences.

Solution: Turn the learning sensitive to psycho-physiological traits of the subject under assessment when available. We found that the inclusion of the relative score for the four Myers-Briggs types[3] was found to increase the accuracy of learning models.

For lazy learners, the simple inclusion of these traits as features is sufficient. We observed an increased accuracy in k-nearest neighbors, which tends to select responses from subjects with related profile.

A simple strategy for non-lazy learners is to partition data by traits, and to learn one model for each trait. Emotion recognition is done by integrating the results of the models with the profile of the testing subject. This integration can recur to a weighted voting scheme, where weights essentially depend on the score obtained for each assessed trait.

A more robust strategy is to learn a tree structure with classification models in the leafs, where a branching decision is associated with trait values that are correlated with heightened response differences for a specific emotion.

---

[3] http://www.myersbriggs.org/.

Table 2. State-of-the-art on existing feature-based models to mine physiological signals

Processing [5,13,24,28]	*Goal*: remove contaminations (noise, interferences and artefacts) *Methods*: segmentation; discard of initial and end signal bands; smoothing filters; low-pass filters such as Adaptive, Elliptic or Butterworth; baseline subtraction; normalization; and discretization techniques
Feature extraction [7,12,17]	*Goal*: extract expressive features, including statistical (mean, deviation, kurtosis), temporal (rise and recovery time), frequency-based and temporal-frequent (geometric analysis, multiscale sample entropy, sub-band spectra) *Methods*: rectangular tonic-phasic windows; moving and sliding features (as mean, median and deviation); transformations (Fourier, wavelet, empirical, Hilbert, singular-spectrum); principal, independent and linear component analysis; projection pursuit; auto-associative networks; multidim. scaling; and self-organizing maps
Feature selection [3,12]	*Goal*: remove features without significant correlation with the emotion under assessment (to improve the space exploitation) *Methods*: sequential forward/backward selection, sequential floating search, branch-and-bound search, principal component analysis, Fisher projection, classifiers (e.g. decision tress, Bayesian networks), Davies-Bouldin index, and analysis of variance methods
Recognition [12,20,21]	*Goal*: classify emotions using the selected features *Methods*: wide-variety of deterministic and probabilistic learners including: k-nearest neighbours, regression trees, random forests, Bayesian networks, support vector machines, canonical correlation and linear discriminant analysis, neural networks, and Marquardt-back propagation

#6: Refine the learning models based on the complexity of emotion expression

Problem: A single emotion-evocative stimulus can elicit small-to-large groups of significantly different physiological responses. A simple generalization of each set of responses leads to poor models.

Solution: Create multiple sub-models for emotions with varying physiological expressions. Both rule-based models, such as random forests, and lazy learners implicitly accommodate this behavior.

Generative models need to be further refined when the emission probabilities of the underlying lattices for a specific emotion do not have a strong convergence. When HMMs are adopted, it is crucial to change the architecture to add an alternative path with a new hidden automaton.

For non-generative models, it is crucial to understand when the model needs to be further refined. This can be done by analyzing the variances of features per emotion or by clustering responses per emotion with a non-fixed number of clusters.

Not only these strategies can improve the emotion recognition rates, but also the characterization of physiological responses per emotion. Consider the case where the learned HMMs are used as a pattern descriptor. Without further separation of different expressions for each emotion, the generative models per emotion would be more prone to error and only reveal generic behavior.

#7: Affect the models to the conditions of the experimental setting

Problem: the properties of the emotion recognition task varies with different settings, such as discrete vs. prolonged stimuli, user-dependent vs. independent studies, univariate vs. multivariate signals.

Solution: The selection and parameterization of classification models should be guided by the experimental conditions. Below we introduced three examples derived from our analysis. First, the influence of sub-peak analysis (principle #2) for emotion recognition should have a higher weight for prolonged stimuli. Second, user-dependent studies are particularly well described by flexible sequential behavior (principle #3). Third, multivariate analysis should be performed in an integrated fashion whenever possible. Common generative models, such as HMMs and dynamic Bayesian networks, are able to model multivariate signals.

Additionally, we found that both the inclusion of other experimental properties (such as interaction annotations) and of the perception of the subject regarding the interaction (assessed recurring to post-surveys) can guide the learning of the target emotion recognition models.

3.2   Methodology

Relying on the introduced seven principles, we propose a novel methodology for emotion recognition and description from physiological signals[4]. Figure 2 illustrates its main steps. Emotion recognition combines the traditional feature-based classification with the results provided from sequence learners and is centered on two expressive representations: *(i)* SAX to normalize individual differences while still preserving overall response pattern, and on *(ii)* local angles to enhance the local sub-peaks of a response. Additionally, emotion characterization is accomplished using both feature-based descriptors (mean and variance of the most discriminative features) and the transition lattices generated by sequence learners.

In the presence of background knowledge, that is, when each instance $(\vec{y}, a_1, ..., a_n, c)$ has $n \geq 1$, prior decisions can be made. Exemplifying, in the presence of psychophysiological traits correlated with varying expression of a specific emotion, the target model can be further decomposed to reduce the complexity of the task.

Complementary, iterative refinements over the learned model can be made when feature-based models rely on features with high variances or when the generative models do not have strong convergence criteria for a specific emotion.

---

[4] Software available in http://web.ist.utl.pt/rmch/research/software/eda.

4 Results

The proposed principles and methodology resulted from an evaluation of advanced data mining and signal processing concepts using a tightly-controlled lab study[5]. More than 200 signals were collected for each physiological modality from both human-to-human and human-to-robot affective interactions. Four physiological modalities – electrodermal activity (EDA), facial expression, skin temperature and 3-dimensional body motion – were monitored using Affectiva technology. Although the conveyed results are mainly centered on electrodermal activity and temperature, previous work from the authors on the use of facial expression to recognize emotion during affective games adds supporting evidence to the relevance of the listed principles [16].

Eight different stimuli, 5 emotion-centered stimuli and 3 others (captured during periods of strong physical effort, concentration and resting), were presented to each subject. A survey was used to categorize the profile of the participants according to the Myers-Briggs type indicator.

The properties of this undertaken experiment are detailed in Table 3. An alternative experiment, interactive chess-playing with iCat robot, with observations that also support the proposed seven principles is detailed in [16].

Statistical and geometric features were extracted from the raw, SAX and local-angle representations. Feature selection was performed using statistical analysis of variance (ANOVA). The selected feature-based classifiers were adopted from WEKA software [8], and the HMMs from HMM-WEKA extension (codified according to Bishop (2006)). SAX and local angle representations were implemented using Java (JVM version 1.6.0-24) and the following results were computed using an Intel Core i5 2.80GHz with 6GB of RAM.

Principles #1 and #2. To assess the impact of dealing with individual differences and informative subtle variations of the signals, we evaluate emotion recognition scores under SAX and local-angle representations using feature-driven models. The score is accuracy, the ability to correctly label an unlabeled signal (i.e. to identify the underline emotion from 5 emotions). Accuracy was computed using a 10 cross-fold validation over the ~200 collected electrodermal signals. Figure 3 synthesizes the results.

The isolated use of electrodermal features from the raw signal (tonic and phasic skin conductivity, maximum amplitude, rising and recovering time) and of statistical features extracted from SAX and local-angle representations leads to an accuracy near 50 % (against 20 % when using a random model). The integration of these features results in an improvement of 10pp to near 60 %. Additionally, accuracy improves when features from skin temperature are included.

Logistic learners, which use regressions on the real-valued features to affect the probability score of each emotion, were the best feature-based models for this experiment. When no feature selection method is applied, Bayesian nets are an attractive alternative. Despite the differences between human-to-human and

---

[5] scripts, data and statistical sheets available in http://web.ist.utl.pt/rmch/research/software/eda.

Table 3. Structural aspects of the conducted experiment.

Physiological signals	30 participants, with ages equally distributed between 19 and 24, were randomly divided in two groups, R and H. Subjects from group R interacted with the NAO robot (http://www. aldebaran-robotics.com) using a wizard-of-Oz setting. The behavior of NAO was expressively implemented and affective synthesized speeches recorded according to a flexible script. Participants from group H interacted with an human agent, an actor with a structured and flexible script
Emotion-evocative stimuli	Empathy (following common practices in speech tone and body approach), expectation (possibility of gaining an additional reward), positive-surprise (unexpected attribution of a significant incremental reward), stress (impossible riddle to solve in a short time to maintain the incremental reward) and frustration (self-responsible loss of the initial and incremental rewards)
Experimental conditions	The stimuli were presented in the same order in every experience; 6–8 minutes was provided between two stimulus to neutralize the subject emotional state and remove the stress related with the experimental expectations; 30-minutes warm-up period was included where subjects solved tests requiring a medium-to-high level of attention; the adopted reward for all subjects was a pair of cinema tickets-offer and the potential additional reward was a Nintendo-Wii; the states of very high and very low arousal were captured to normalize the features; the experiment was conducted in an appealing context to not desensitize the subject; the experience was recorded and documented to be audited and reproduced

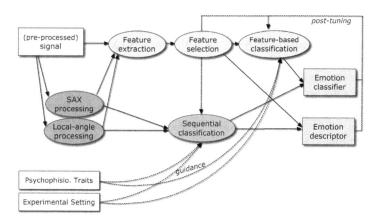

Fig. 2. Proposed methodology for emotion recognition & description from physiological signals

human-to-robot settings, classifiers are still able to recognize emotions when mixing the cases. For instance, kNN tends to select the features from a sole scenario when $k < 4$, while C4.5 trees have dedicated branches for each scenario (Fig. 3).

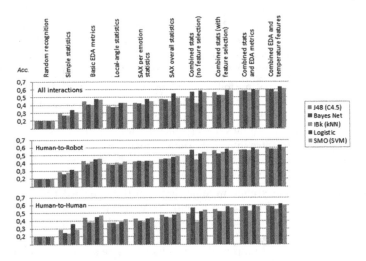

Fig. 3. Emotion recognition accuracy (out of 5 emotions) using feature-driven models

These accuracy levels also reveal the adequacy of emotion description models that rely on centroid and dispersion metrics over the most discriminative features.

Additionally, to understand the relevance of features extracted from SAX and local-angle representations to differentiate emotions under assessment, one-way ANOVA tests were applied with the Tukey post-hoc analysis. A significance of 5 % was considered for the Levene's test of variance homogeneity, ANOVA and Tukey tests. Both features derived from the raw, SAX and local-angle electrodermal signals were considered. A representative set of electrodermal features able to separate emotions is synthesized in Table 4.

Gradient plus centroid metrics from SAX signals can be adopted to separate negative emotions. Dispersion metrics from local-angle representations differentiate positive emotions. Rise time and response amplitude can be used to isolate specific emotions, and statistical features, such as median and distortion, to predict the affective valence. Kurtosis, which reveals the flatness of the response's major peak, and features derived from the temperature signal were also able to differentiate emotions with significance using the proposed representations.

Principles #3 and #4. In our experimental setting, the inclusion of sequential behavior leads to an increase of accuracy levels nearly 10pp. The output of HMMs were, additionally, combined the output of probabilistic feature-based classifiers (logistic learners were the choice). Table 5 discloses the results when adopting

Table 4. Features with potential to discriminate emotions

Features (with strongest statistical significance to differentiate emotions' sets)	Separated emotions
Accentuated *dispersion* metrics (such as the mean square error) from the SAX and local-angle signals	Positive: empathy, expectation and surprise
Median (relevant to quantify the sustenance of peaks), *distortion* and *recovery time* from SAX signals	Positive from negative from neutral emotions
Gradient (revealing long-term sympathetic activation by measuring the EDA baseline changed) and *centroid* metrics from SAX signals	Fear from frustration
Rise time	Empathy from others
Response amplitude	Surprise from others

HMMs with alternative architectures for approximately 30 signals per emotion (empathy, expectation, surprise, stress, frustration).

Table 5. Accuracy of sequence learners to correctly classify an emotion out of 5 emotions (recognition accuracy) and to correctly discard the 3 least probable emotions (discrimination accuracy)

			Electrodermal SAX signal	Including local-angle	Including temperature	Including EDA metrics
HMM (fully-connected architecture)	Recognition accuracy	All	0.40	0.42	0.46	0.67
		Robot	0.39	0.41	0.44	0.66
		Human	0.39	0.42	0.45	0.67
	Discrimination accuracy	All	0.86	0.88	0.89	–
		Robot	0.87	0.88	0.91	–
		Human	0.86	0.88	0.90	–
HMM (left-to-right architecture [22])	Recognition accuracy	All	0.43	0.44	0.48	0.71
		Robot	0.42	0.43	0.47	0.71
		Human	0.41	0.44	0.47	0.69
	Discrimination accuracy	All	0.87	0.88	0.90	–
		Robot	0.87	0.89	0.90	–
		Human	0.87	0.88	0.89	–

Interestingly, the learned HMMs are highly prone to accurately neglect 3 emotion labels that do not fit in the learned behavior. In particular, left-to-right HMM architectures are particularly well-suited to mine SAX-based signals. Note, additionally, that left-to-right architectures are a good emotion descriptor due to the high interpretability of the most probable behavior of the signal when disclosing

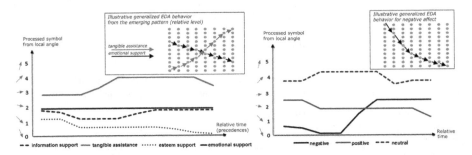

Fig. 4. Emerging sequential patterns of fixed length the different supportive behavior of the robot (information-centered tangible, esteem, emotional) and different affective states (negative, neutral, positive) of the participants during interactive chess-play (details in [16]).

the most probable emissions along the main path. Similar architectures can be implemented by controlling the initial transition and emission probabilities.

Although the local-angle representation is not as critical as SAX for sequential learning, its weighted use for emotion recognition and discrimination has a positive impact in the accuracy levels.

The why behind the success of adopting HMMs with SAX or local angle representations for emotion recognition resides on their ability to:

– detect flexible behavior, such as peak-sustaining values and fluctuations that are hardly measured by features;
– cope with individual differences (with the scaling being done with respect to all stimuli, to the target stimulus, to all subjects or to subject-specific responses);
– cope with subtle but meaningful variations of the signal;
– deal with lengthy responses (by increasing the number of hidden states);
– capture either a smoothed behavior or a more delineated behavior by controlling the signal cardinality.

The relevance of mining prototype sequential behavior per emotion can be also supported through the retrieval of frequent precedences. In one of our previous studies [16], where physiological signals were collected from children engaging with the *i*Cat robot during affective chess games, we identified significantly differential behavior (extracted using sequential pattern mining). In Fig. 4 we extract emerging electrodermal behavior for the monitored children in response to: *(1)* different supportive behavior adopted by *i*Cat, and *(2)* different affective states of the participant (labeled by the *i*Cat). Illustrating, the affect-oriented behavior (esteem and emotional support) caused lower levels of EDA, suggesting better efficacy on relaxing the participant. Also, states with neutral affection, where the participant is neither moving nor conveying affective facial expressions, have growing EDA as they seem to be associated with states of high concentration, attention and reasoning.

Table 6. Influence of subjects' profile on EDA responses

Myers-Briggs type	*Correlated features* ([+] positive correlation; [−] negative correlation)
Extrovert-introvert	[+] Dispersion metrics of SAX signal
	[−] Centroid metrics of SAX signal
	[−] Response amplitude
Sensing-intuition	[−] Dispersion metrics of raw and SAX signal
	[−] Dispersion metrics of local-angles
	[−] Rise time
Feeling-thinking	[+] Median and dispersion metrics of SAX signal
	[−] Declive and centroid metrics of local-angles
	[−] Rise time
Judging-perceiving	[−] Centroid metrics of raw signal
	[−] Dispersion metrics of SAX signal
	[+] Response amplitude

Principle #5. Pearson correlations were tested to correlate the physiological expression with the subjects profile. This analysis, illustrated in Table 6, shows that their inclusion can be a critical input to guide the learning task. A positive (negative) correlation means that higher (lower) values for the assessed feature are related with a polarization towards either the extrovert, sensing, feeling or perceiving type.

We can observe, for instance, that responses from sensors and feelers are quicker, while extroverts have a more instable signal (higher dispersion) although less intense (lower amplitude).

The insertion of the relative score for the four Myers-Briggs types was found to increase the accuracy of IBk, who tend to select responses from subjects with related profile. Also, for non-lazy probabilistic learners, four data partitions were created, with the first separating extroverts from introverts and so on. One model was learned for each profile. Recognition for a test instance now relies on the equally weighted combined output of each model, which result in an increased accuracy of 2–3pp. Although the improvement seems to be subtle, note that the split of instances hampers the learning of these models since we it relies on a reduced number of signals.

Principle #6. The analysis of the variance of key features and of the learned generative models per emotion provide critical insights for further adaptations of the learning task. For instance, the variance of rising time across subjects for positive-surprise was observed to be high due to the fact that some subjects tend to experience a short period of distrust. The inclusion of similar features in logistic model trees, where a feature can be tested multiple times using different values, revealed that they tend to be often selected, and, therefore, should not be removed due to their high variance.

Another illustrative observation was the weak convergence of the Markov model for empathy due to its idiosyncratic expression. Under this knowledge, we adapted the left-to-right architecture to include three main paths. After learning this new model, we verified a heightened convergence of the model for each one of the empathy paths, revealing three distinct forms of physiological expression and, consequently, an improved recognition rate.

Principle #7. We performed additional tests to understand the impact of the experimental conditions on the physiological expression of emotions. First, we performed a t-test to assess the influence of features derived from the signal collected during all the affective interaction (without partitions by stimulus) on the adopted type of interaction (human-to-human vs. human-to-robot). Results over the SAX representation show that human-to-human interactions (in comparison to human-to-robot) have significantly: *(i)* a higher median (revealing an increased ability to sustain peaks), and *(ii)* higher values of dispersion and kurtosis (revealing heightened emotional response).

Second, we studied the impact of the subjects' perception on the experiment by correlating signal features with the answers to a survey made at the end of the interaction. Bivariate Pearson correlation between a set of scored variables assessed in the final survey and physiological features was performed at a 5 % significance level. Table 7 synthesizes the most significant correlations found. They include positive correlation of local-angle dispersion (revealing changes in the gradient) with intensity, felt influence and perceived intention; positive correlation of SAX dispersion (revealing heightened variations from the baseline) with the perceived empathy, confidence and trust; quicker rise time for heightened perceived optimism; and higher amplitude of responses for heightened felt influence and low levels of pleasure.

Table 7. Influence of subject perception in the physiological expression of emotions

Origin	*Correlations* with higher statistical significance
Local-angle features	[+] Dispersion metrics with the felt intensity, the understanding of the agent's intention, and his level of influence on felt emotions
SAX-based features	[+] Dispersion metrics with the perceived empathy, trust and confidence of the agent
Computed metrics	[+] Amplitude with the perceived agent influence
	[-] Amplitude with the felt pleasure
	[-] Rise time with the perceived positivism on the agent's attitude

In a complementary note, the results collected from one of our previous studies [16] where physiological signals were monitored during affective chess-playing with a robot, also suggest that statistical properties of the signal are correlated with the participants' perception of the interaction. In particular, engagement, motivation and attention (surveyed through questionnaires) were found to be discriminated with statistical significance by physiological features.

These two observations motivate the need to turn the learning models sensitive to additional information related with experimental conditions and with the subject perception and expectations. Their inclusion as new features in feature-based learners resulted in a generalized improved accuracy (3–5pp).

5 Conclusion

This work provides seven key principles on how to recognize and describe emotions during affective interactions from physiological signals. These principles aim to overcome the limitations of existing emotion-centered methods to mine signals. We propose the use of expressive signal representations to correct individual differences and account for subtle variations, as well as the integration of generative and feature-based views.

We demonstrate the relevance of using specific knowledge of the learned models and annotations related with the experimental setting to improve the learning task. Additionally, we show that psychological traits can guide this task by correcting profile-driven differences, opening a new direction on how to measure affective interactions.

A new methodology was proposed to coherently integrate these principles. This methodology provides a roadmap for the combined application of the seven principles and for the development of new methods.

We presented initial empirical evidence that supports the utility for each one the enumerated principles. In particular, we observed that the adoption of techniques to incorporate the seven principles can improve emotion recognition rates by 20pp.

Promoting the quality of classification and descriptive models of emotions opens a new door for the psycho-physiological study and real-time monitoring of affective interactions. Therefore, in a context where the use of non-intrusive wearable sensors is rapidly increasing, this paper establishes solid foundations for upcoming contributions on this critical field of research.

Acknowledgments. This article is an extended version of our previous work [10]. This work is supported by Fundação para a Ciência e Tecnologia under the project PEst-OE/EEI/LA0021/2013 and PhD grant SFRH/BD/ 75924/2011, and by the project EMOTE from the EU 7thFramework Program (FP7/2007–2013). The authors would like to thank: Tiago Ribeiro for implementing the robots' behavior with sharp expressiveness, Iolanda Leite and Ivo Capelo for their support during the preparation and execution of the experiments, and Arvid Kappas for his contributions on the design of the experiments.

References

1. Andreassi, J.: Psychophysiology: Human Behavior and Physiological Response. Lawrence Erlbaum, Mahwah (2007)
2. Bishop, C.M.: Pattern Recognition and Machine Learning. Information Science and Statistics. Springer, New York (2006)

3. Bos, D.O.: EEG-based emotion recognition the influence of visual and auditory stimuli. Emotion **57**(7), 1798–1806 (2006)
4. Cacioppo, J., Tassinary, L., Berntson, G.: Handbook of Psychophysiology. Cambridge University Press, New York (2007)
5. Chang, C., Zheng, J., Wang, C.: Based on support vector regression for emotion recognition using physiological signals. In: IJCNN, pp. 1–7 (2010)
6. Ekman, P., Friesen, W.V., O'Sullivan, M., Chan, A., Diacoyanni-Tarlatzis, I., Heider, K., Krause, R., LeCompte, W.A., Pitcairn, T., Ricci-Bitti, P.E., Scherer, K.R., Tomita, M., Tzavaras, A.: Universals and cultural differences in the judgments of facial expressions of emotion. J. Pers. Soc. Psychol. **53**, 712–717 (1988)
7. Haag, A., Goronzy, S., Schaich, P., Williams, J.: Emotion recognition using biosensors: first steps towards an automatic system. In: André, E., Dybkjær, L., Minker, W., Heisterkamp, P. (eds.) ADS 2004. LNCS (LNAI), vol. 3068, pp. 36–48. Springer, Heidelberg (2004)
8. Hall, M., Frank, E., Holmes, G., Pfahringer, B., Reutemann, P., Witten, I.H.: The WEKA data mining software: an update. SIGKDD Explor. Newsl. **11**(1), 10–18 (2009)
9. Henriques, R., Paiva, A.: Descriptive models of emotion: learning useful abstractions from physiological responses during affective interactions. In: PhyCS Special Session on Recognition of Affect Signals from PhysiologIcal Data for Social Robots (OASIS'14). SCITEPRESS, Lisbon (2014)
10. Henriques, R., Paiva, A.: Seven principles to mine flexible behavior from physiological signals for effective emotion recognition and description in affective interactions. In: Physiological Computing Systems (PhyCS'14). SCITEPRESS, Lisbon (2014)
11. Henriques, R., Paiva, A., Antunes, C.: On the need of new methods to mine electrodermal activity in emotion-centered studies. In: Cao, L., Zeng, Y., Symeonidis, A.L., Gorodetsky, V.I., Yu, P.S., Singh, M.P. (eds.) ADMI. LNCS (LNAI), vol. 7607, pp. 203–215. Springer, Heidelberg (2013)
12. Jerritta, S., Murugappan, M., Nagarajan, R., Wan, K.: Physiological signals based human emotion recognition: a review. In: IEEE 7th International Colloquium on Signal Processing and its Applications (CSPA) 2011, pp. 410–415 (2011)
13. Katsis, C., Katertsidis, N., Ganiatsas, G., Fotiadis, D.: Toward emotion recognition in car-racing drivers: a biosignal processing approach. IEEE Trans. Syst. Man Cybern. Syst. Hum. **38**(3), 502–512 (2008)
14. Kulic, D., Croft, E.A.: Affective state estimation for human-robot interaction. Trans. Rob. **23**(5), 991–1000 (2007)
15. Lang, P.: The emotion probe: studies of motivation and attention. Am. Psychol. **50**, 372–372 (1995)
16. Leite, I., Henriques, R., Martinho, C., Paiva, A.: Sensors in the wild: exploring electrodermal activity in child-robot interaction. In: HRI, pp. 41–48. ACM/IEEE (2013)
17. Lessard, C.S.: Signal Processing of Random Physiological Signals. Synthesis Lectures on Biomedical Engineering. Morgan and Claypool Publishers, San Rafael (2006)
18. Lin, J., Keogh, E., Lonardi, S., Chiu, B.: A symbolic representation of time series, with implications for streaming algorithms. In: ACM SIGMOD Workshop on DMKD, pp. 2–11. ACM, New York (2003)
19. Lin, J., Keogh, E.J., Lonardi, S., Chiu, B.Y.: A symbolic representation of time series, with implications for streaming algorithms. In: Zaki, M.J., Aggarwal, C.C. (eds.) DMKD, pp. 2–11. ACM (2003)

20. Maaoui, C., Pruski, A., Abdat, F.: Emotion recognition for human-machine communication. In: IROS, pp. 1210–1215. IEEE/RSJ (2008)
21. Mitsa, T.: Temporal data mining. In: DMKD. Chapman & Hall/CRC (2009)
22. Murphy, K.: Dynamic Bayesian networks: representation, inference and learning. Ph.D. thesis, UC Berkeley, CS Division (2002)
23. Oatley, K., Keltner, D., Jenkins, J.M.: Understanding Emotions. Blackwell, Cambridge (2006)
24. Petrantonakis, P., Hadjileontiadis, L.: Emotion recognition from EEG using higher order crossings. TITB **14**(2), 186–197 (2010)
25. Picard, R.W.: Affective computing: challenges. Int. J. Hum. Comput. Stud. **59**(1–2), 55–64 (2003)
26. Picard, R.W., Vyzas, E., Healey, J.: Toward machine emotional intelligence: analysis of affective physiological state. IEEE Trans. Pattern Anal. Mach. Intell. **23**(10), 1175–1191 (2001)
27. Rani, P., Liu, C., Sarkar, N., Vanman, E.: An empirical study of machine learning techniques for affect recognition in human-robot interaction. Pattern Anal. Appl. **9**(1), 58–69 (2006)
28. Rigas, G., Katsis, C.D., Ganiatsas, G., Fotiadis, D.I.: A user independent, biosignal based, emotion recognition method. In: Conati, C., McCoy, K., Paliouras, G. (eds.) UM 2007. LNCS (LNAI), vol. 4511, pp. 314–318. Springer, Heidelberg (2007)
29. Villon, O., Lisetti, C.: Toward recognizing individual's subjective emotion from physiological signals in practical application. In: Computer-Based Medical Systems, pp. 357–362 (2007)
30. Vyzas, E.: Recognition of emotional and cognitive states using physiological data. Master's thesis, MIT (1999)
31. Wagner, J., Kim, J., Andre, E.: From physiological signals to emotions: implementing and comparing selected methods for feature extraction and classification. In: ICME, pp. 940–943. IEEE (2005)
32. Wu, C.K., Chung, P.C., Wang, C.J.: Extracting coherent emotion elicited segments from physiological signals. In: WACI, pp. 1–6. IEEE (2011)

A Generic Effort-Based Behavior Description for User Engagement Analysis

Benedikt Gollan[1]([✉]) and Alois Ferscha[2]

[1] Pervasive Computing Applications, Research Studios Austria, Thurngasse 8/20,
1080 Vienna, Austria
benedikt.gollan@researchstudio.at
[2] Institute for Pervasive Computing, Johannes Kepler University,
Altenberger Strasse 69, 4040 Linz, Austria
ferscha@pervasive.jku.at

Abstract. Human interaction is to a large extent based on implicit, unconscious behavior and the related body language. In this article, we propose 'Directed Effort' a generic description of human behavior suitable as user engagement and interest input for higher level human-computer interaction applications. Research from behavioral and psychological sciences is consulted for the creation of an attention model which is designed to represent the engagement of people towards generic objects in public spaces. The functionality of this behavior analysis approach is demonstrated in a prototypical implementation to present the potential of the presented meta-level description of behavior.

Keywords: Automatic behavior analysis · Movement tracking · Pattern recognition · Estimation of engagement

1 Introduction

Behavior and body language are crucial aspects of any kind of interaction between humans. Besides the pure entropy of information which can be represented bit-wise, it is the subtle indicators like the sarcastic tone of voice, the rolling of the eyes or the impatient tapping of the foot through which we transmit the majority of the information which is necessary to successfully interpret messages. Human interaction is largely based on the meticulous interpretation of meta-information for which, even among humans, experts are rare. This poses an immense challenge to all researchers and designers of human-computer interaction systems that aim at creating natural and intuitive user interfaces, trying to best possible generate a human-like interaction quality experience in human-computer interaction systems.

Human behavior encompasses any observable physical activity. Yet, the description of behavior not only has to cover different aspects of behavior depending on the respective field of application, but can also imply many different layers of abstraction. These can range from a technical analysis of body pose based on

© Springer-Verlag Berlin Heidelberg 2014
H.P. da Silva et al. (Eds.): PhyCS 2014, LNCS 8908, pp. 157–169, 2014.
DOI: 10.1007/978-3-662-45686-6_10

joint coordinates and orientations to a higher-level interpretation of body language, or from the pure analysis of movement speed data to an interpretation of underlying motivations and intentions. An ideal representation of behavior will of course include all behavioral aspects and layers, whereas actual applications and implementations will set limitations to what is necessary, useful and technically feasible.

As human interaction is largely based on the interpretation of human behavior, we need to create representations of behavior which allow further interpretations of intentions that go beyond explicit user input. In this work, we try to approach such a potential higher level description which may be applicable to represent the orientation and level of human commitment, engagement and interest. For this purpose, we propose a generic meta-level description of behavior which is designed to be generally valid, generic, independent from sensor technology, and quantifiable to be suitable for various human-computer interaction applications.

1.1 Related Work

Commitment and behavior have often been approached from different scientific fields which resulted in numerous strategies towards specific aspects and effects related to behavior, commitment and attention. Elaborate surveys on human behavior analysis have been composed by Ji et al. [12] and Candamo et al. [5].

Concentrating on technical realizations, the implementations can be divided into the already indicated categories of action or activity recognition and a semantic representation of behavior. Activity analysis can be covered by template-based or state-space-based approaches. Employing templates, Bobick and Davis [3] first used *motion energy images* and *motion history images* to represent and categorize activities. Blank et al. [2] extracted the 3D silhouette of people to enable a fast and robust classification of activities. State-space approaches interpret human behavior as a state machine with different postures as states. These are often represented via Hidden-Markov-Models (HMMs) [18, 21].

Semantic descriptions of behavior have gained momentum lately. The importance of body orientation in human interaction is investigated by Hietanen [9] with the result that head and upper body orientation are vital components which nonverbally transfer the aspect of engagement in an interaction. Guevara and Umemuro [8] implemented a behavior analysis to infer on psychological states, finding that walking velocity and motion load are suitable for predicting sadness or neutral states of mind.

Usually, in human-computer interaction human-computer interaction research, commitment is interpreted as equivalent to visual focus and no further attention model is integrated. Smith et al. [22] created a head tracking and gaze estimation system which detects whether passing people are actually watching a shop window. Yakiyama et al. [24] estimate commitment levels towards target objects via a laser sensor and on the basis of computed distance, basic orientation and movement speed. According to Knudsen [14] orienting movements are used to optimize the resolution of (visual) information about the object.

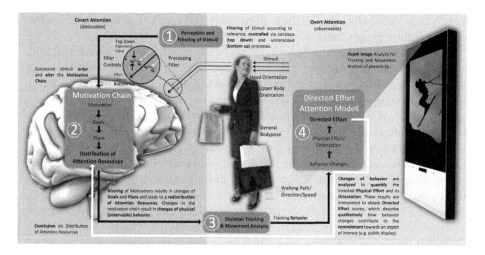

Fig. 1. Schematic illustration of the intrinsic and exterior processes of behavior control. (1) Incoming stimuli are filtered according to top down and bottom up processes (SEEV model [23]). (2) Succeeding stimuli enter and alter the Motivation Chain and influence the distribution of Attention Resources. (3) Realization of Plans expresses in observable behavior. (4) Behavior changes can be tracked, quantified and interpreted.

2   The Creation and Control of Behavior

Human behavior addresses any observable physical activity of the individual. To enable a successful interpretation, it is essential to understand basic underlying behavioral mechanisms. This chapter will describe a model derived from psychology and behavior research of how behavior is motivated, controlled and initialized.

Following Bongers [4] and Dijksterhuis [7], behavior is controlled via a sequential motivation chain (Fig. 1): Input stimuli are processed and filtered regarding their value, importance and salience. The successive stimuli compete with already existing *Motivations* for their realization. The result of this competition is a set of prioritized *Goals*, that describe the intrinsic, often unconscious intentions of a person. These cannot be assessed from the outside and may be as simple as 'being hungry', or complex structures which can not be verbalized at all. To actually achieve these abstract *Goals*, we make concrete *Plans* like navigating to the next restaurant, to satisfy the underlying motivation. Finally, the actual realization of these plans leads to the execution of observable physical behavior.

With outward behavior visualizing and representing inner states, a thorough analysis of pyhsical behavior holds great potential for a suitable analysis of the level and even orientation of inner commitment. Elementary changes in the motivation chain, e.g. triggered by sudden extrinsic stimuli (siren, etc.) will cause a sequence of re-prioritization of Goals and Plans and finally result in alterations of physical behavior. Our approach is directed at the observation and interpretation of such behavioral changes, to infer alterations and repriorizations in the unfortunately unobservable motivation chain.

The proposed model correlates very well with existing behavior control findings. Posner [19] investigated the connection between extrinsic behavior, e.g. head turning, eye movements towards selected stimuli and inner processes which describe all completely mental activities. Posner found the relation between covert and overt attention to be not a close but a functional one, showing a 'striking tendency of attention to move to the target prior to an eye movement'. Hoffman [10] showed that, being ordered to direct gaze towards a certain location, one cannot attend objects at a different location. This existence of a neural structural connection between exterior and inner focus was supported by Moore [15], Perry [17] and Rizzolatti [20]. On the other hand, experiments carried out by Hunt and Kingstone [11] indicate that in case of bottom-up controlled, reflexive processes overt and covert attention are strongly related whereas for top-down controlled processes, inferring backwards from eye gaze alone to overt attention is error-prone. The difference between reflexive and voluntary controlled mechanisms is supported by Müller and Rabbitt [16], who detected higher reorientation performances for reflexive reorientation of attentional focus.

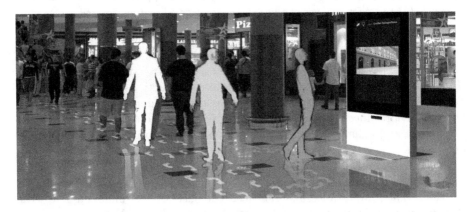

Fig. 2. Different kinds of behavior in a mall scenario when passing a public display. (a, white) Passers-by may not perceive the display at all and show no reaction, (b, yellow) turn their head towards the screen but continuing current general behavior of approaching their destination or (c, green) actually changing the path, investing time and commitment in perceiving the presented information (Color figure online).

3   Effort as Key-Parameter for Behavior Analysis

Having a model of how behavior is generated, the next step is to find a suitable representation which is characteristic for all kinds of behavior and especially describes changes of behavior in a qualitative and quantitative way.

Every alteration of existing plans and accordingly of current behavior is characterized by its demand for a certain amount of *Mental Effort*, which includes the process of filtering stimuli input and deciding to commit to a source of information and consequently a rescheduling of future tasks. Furthermore, it requires *Physical Effort*, '*an important concept, ... required to access different sources of information, using whatever mechanism is necessary: eyes, head, body, hands or even the walking feet*' [23], to actually alter physical behavior.

In this context, the principle of the economy of movement represents a crucial aspect. As Bitgood states: '*To overcome the economy of movement motivation,.., the perceived benefits of approaching an attractive object must outweigh the perceived cost of the effort*' [1]. Generally, people tend to optimize their behavior concerning energy consumption and effort, physical or mental, as '*excessive mental effort, like excessive physical effort, generally produces an unpleasant state that is to be avoided. Hence, people tend to be inherently effort conserving, particularly when placed in high demanding environments...*' [23]. Consequently, we assume that one will stick to his current comportment until given valid reason to change, thus evading unnecessary investment of effort.

To give an example, in spatial contexts, behavior control is influenced by the effort which is necessary to access information sources. This physical effort involves all overt processes from eye movement, over body posture to movement parameters. Kahneman states that '*because of the connection between effort and arousal, physiological measures of arousal can be used to measure the exertion of effort*' [13]. According to Knudsen [14] Orienting Movements are used to optimize the resolution of (visual) information about the object. To demonstrate these principles, a sample scenario of a person moving through a shopping mall is displayed in Fig. 2. Passing a public display, there are different behaviors that can be adopted. In the sample scenario, the described options (a)–(c) differ in the amount of energy and time which are invested to engage with the display and the presented content. As can be observed, the more effort is invested the higher will be the commitment to the object.

Bringing it all together as illustrated in Fig. 1, in the complete process of (i) filtering stimuli, over (ii) alteration of the motivation chain to the (iii) allocation of attention resources and finally to the (iv) execution of related plans to satisfy underlying motivations, it is named Effort which represents the critical threshold of whether attention resources are assigned and behavior is changed. At the same time it represents an observable indicator of physical commitment to a source of information. With effort being (not the only but) such an important regulating factor in behavior control, we propose physical effort as the basis for a generic and generally applicable higher level representation of behavior.

4   Behavior Analysis Framework

Providing a valid measurement of behavior, demands three important elements: (a) measuring directly significant target behavior, (b) measuring a relevant dimension of target behavior and (c) ensuring that the data is representative for the given use-case [6]. In this chapter, a behavior measure framework is proposed based on interpreting behavioral changes which tries to best possibly match these prerequisites.

To approach an actual implementation, changes of behavior need to be detected, quantified and evaluated. We assume an interaction system with any kind and number of sensor-based tracking system(s) (cameras, distance sensors, depth sensors, etc.) with which behavioral data can be collected. The collected behavior data depends on the choice of sensor and application scenario and may include any measurable data that describes movement in a characteristic way like skeleton joint coordinates, gaze direction, etc.

Our proposed framework (Fig. 3) defines four important variables, which are behavioral parameters $b_i(t)$, Effort $e_i(t)$, Effect $f_i(t)$ and Directed Effort $DE(t)$.

$$b_i(t) = s(i, t) \tag{1}$$
$$e_i(t) = \Delta(b_i(t), B_i(t_0; t-1))) \tag{2}$$
$$f_i(t) = \Phi(b_i(t), \vec{x}) \tag{3}$$
$$DE(t) = \sum \alpha_i \cdot e_i(t) \cdot f_i(t) \tag{4}$$

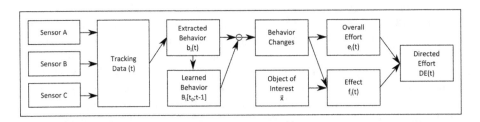

Fig. 3. Visualization of behavior analysis framework components. Tracking data is collected from sensor(s). Feature extraction algorithms provide behavior data which is used to calculate reference behavior and current behavior changes. The changes of behavior are processed to effort scores and evaluated in relation to the location of the object of interest to obtain effect information. Finally, effort and effect are combined to a single expressive feature called Directed Effort which describes the level of engagement of behavior changes to an object of interest.

Behavior parameters b_i (1) describe the sensor data $s(t)$ extracted to exclusively describe a single aspect of behavior i. These could range from movement speed, orientation or location of single body joints to a emitted volume of whole groups of people. The selection of these behavioral features heavily depends on the application and choice of sensor. For later evaluation of the data, it is necessary to best possible isolate the characteristic parameters of the aspired behavior parameter in the feature extraction process. Please note, the behavior parameters may range from mere numeric to directed dimensions like vectors, angles, etc. Due to this variety, the notation has been confined to an abstract placeholder b_i.

The extracted behavior data is used to calculate changes in behavior individually for each behavior parameter per frame t. For this purpose, training data B_i is collected to describe recent reference behavior which is used to detect the amount of alterations. The process of calculating the amount of effort $e_i(t)$ which is required to execute the detected change of behavior (2) is represented via Δ (5). In this function, effort is represented via a percental representation in relation to the maximal possible change of behavior for the respective behavior parameter. E.g., turning the head with an angle of $20°$ and assuming a maximum turn of $180°$ would result in an effort of $20°/180° = 11,1\%$ for the behavioral parameter of head turn. In spite of the issue of defining these maximum values, this process provides a normalized level of effort scores throughout completely unrelated parameters of behavior, making them comparable.

$$\Delta(b_i(t), B_i[t_0;\ t-1]) = \frac{b_i(t) - B_i(t)}{b_{i,max}} \tag{5}$$

These effort scores e_i represent the overall and unevaluated invested effort scores. Accumulating over i would deliver the overall amount of invested effort. Yet, the proposed isolated representation of the effort per behavior parameter is necessary for the following evaluation of the orientation and effect of the invested effort. Assuming that all behavior changes are causally determined, our approach tries to interpret the effect of the detected behavior to deduce the source of the behavioral change and thus draw conclusions on the underlying motivations.

Given the vast amount of potential objects of interest and the high possibility that the actual sources of the behavior change are unknown and outside of the observable area, the evaluation has to be restricted to distinct objects. This restriction will not allow a general identification of sources of interest but at least enables the observation and evaluation of distinct, single targets. By defining the location $\vec{x}$ of an object of interest (OOI) in the observed scene, it is possible to analyze the effect f_i of the change on potential commitment to this OOI. The evaluation of the behavior data (Eq. 3) in relation to the location of a reference OOI is represented by Φ (6). Again, this function needs to be accustomed to the specific behavior parameter and a percental representation is proposed.

$$\Phi(e_i(t), \vec{x}) = \frac{\vec{b_i}\,(t, \vec{x})}{b_{i,opt}} \tag{6}$$

As a final step, extracted information concerning the amount and the effect of the invested Physical Effort are combined into a single expressive value called *Directed Effort* (4) which represents the effective invested Effort which is has been evaluated as contributive regarding potential OOI. In other words, Directed Effort scores describe how much effort which is directed at a specific object, has been invested. The already calculated values $e_i(t)$ and $f_i(t)$ hold the amount and effect of the respective behavior parameters i. To combine them to a single expressive score, the products of the corresponding effort and effect scores are accumulated and weighted with a factor α_i. This weighting again depends on the application scenario and choice of parameters. By interpreting these Direct Effort scores, we hope to be able to draw conclusions on the distribution of attention resources which has evoked the observed behavior.

5   Exemplary Implementation

To demonstrate the functionality of the proposed framework, a sample implementation is described in the following. A public display scenario has been selected, in which the commitment of passers-by to the displayed content is supposed to be investigated. To enable behavior analysis, a large-scale public display has been equipped with a depth sensor which allows an accurate tracking of body pose and extraction of movement features of passers-by.

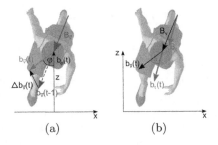

Fig. 4. (a) Visualization of behavior parameters b_v, b_φ and (b) b_τ.

First, the aspired behavior parameters b_i need to be identified and defined. In the given scenario, behavior can be unraveled into the three existing degrees of freedom of movement which are *movement direction, body orientation* and *velocity*.

Body orientation is set identical to head orientation, as it turned out to be the orientation component of the highest relevance and the best tracking results in our implementation. The effort component which derives from movement direction and body orientation is calculated as the difference of the detected current angles b_τ and b_φ (Fig. 4) to learned current reference values B_τ and B_φ. In this application, the 'learned' components B_i are implemented as an exponentially decreasing low-pass filter (10). Finally the alteration is set in relation to the maximum change per parameter, which are $\pm 180°$ for movement direction and $\pm 90°$ for head orientation.

To calculate the effort invested in a change of speed, acceleration values b_v can be analyzed. Yet, here a different approach is followed, since relation to a theoretical maximal acceleration value does not adequately describe real circumstances. In this case, an acceleration from $5\frac{m}{s}$ to $10\frac{m}{s}$ would result in the same effort as an increase from $15\frac{m}{s}$ to $20\frac{m}{s}$, although in the first case the speed has been doubled. This is why a different percentaged representation has been chosen which describes the percentaged change in relation to recent velocity. Note, that only effort from behavior changes are analyzed at this point, although of course, maintaining a high speed will involve immense physical effort. The inclusion of these constant aspects of effort are part of current research for the generalization and enlargement of the framework.

$$e_v(t) = \frac{b_v(t)}{B_v} \tag{7}$$

$$e_\varphi(t) = \frac{|(b_\varphi(t) - B_\varphi)|}{90} \tag{8}$$

$$e_\tau(t) = \frac{|e_\tau(t)| - B_\tau}{180} \tag{9}$$

$$B_i = \frac{1}{30} \cdot \sum_{n=0}^{30} \frac{1}{n} \cdot b_i(t - n) \tag{10}$$

To analyze the effect of the invested effort towards the display location, the orientation of the behavioral changes has to be evaluated in relation to the location of the display, which results in a measure of the contributivity of the detected activities to the display location. E.g. a person making a turn of 90° will always result in the same detected physical effort no matter where in the scene the activity took place. But is the interpretation of the orientation towards the display which elevates the detected physical effort from a pure mathematical description of activity to an expressive representation of potential commitment, which is Directed Effort. It enables us to interpret whether activities are directed towards or away from the display, bringing the person to a more or less attentive state.

To evaluate the acceleration parameter $b_v(t)$ (Fig. 5(a)) a rule-based evaluation function ϕ_v is selected. First, the absolute effective fraction of the acceleration vector $\vec{a}$ to the display location is analyzed to evaluate to what degree the activity is related to the display. Second, a rule-based evaluation of the contributivity is applied which relies on the assumption that any activity which increases the stay in the range of the display or improves the perception of the display is considered as contributive. Hence, all deceleration and movement into the display sector are interpreted as positive effect, whereas all accelerations which are directed away from the display are evaluated as negative effect (13).

$$\Phi_v(t, \vec{x}) = \rho_v(t) \cdot b_{v,f}(t) \tag{11}$$

$$b_{v,x}(t) = \frac{\vec{x} \bullet \overrightarrow{b_v(t)}}{|\vec{x}|^2} \cdot \vec{x} \tag{12}$$

$$\rho_v(t) = \begin{cases} 1, & \text{if } b_v(t) < 0 \ || \ w[t] \ \leq \epsilon_1, \epsilon_2, \\ -1, & \text{else.} \end{cases} \tag{13}$$

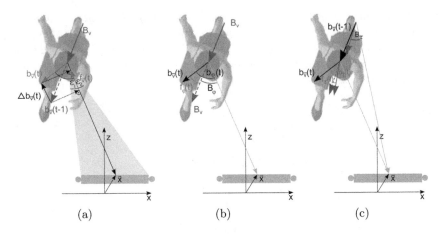

Fig. 5. Computation of the Effect of (a) the acceleration $\Delta b_{\vec{v}}(t)$ by computing the component of $f_{\vec{v}}(t)$ that is directed at the object (orthogonal projection of $\Delta b_{\vec{v}}(t)$ onto the direct connection to the object location), (b) $b_\varphi(t)$ by the change of movement angle towards the object and (c) $b_\tau(t)$ by change of orientation angle $f_\tau(t)$ towards the object.

Considering the effect of variations in movement direction and orientation, changes are considered beneficial, if the movement causes the angle towards the display location to decrease (Eqs. 14 and 15). Again, the effect scores are percentaged in relation to the maximal value.

$$\Phi_f(t) = \frac{(B_{\varphi,x} - b_{\varphi,x}(t))}{180} \tag{14}$$

$$\Phi_\tau(t) = \frac{(B_{\tau,x} - b_{\tau,x}(t))}{180} \tag{15}$$

$$DE = \sum_i \alpha_i \cdot e_i(t) \cdot f_i(t) \tag{16}$$

Bringing it all together, the effort and effect scores are weighted with parameters α_i and accumulated to the final Directed Effort score. The weighting parameters are necessary to create a more life-like distribution of effort scores and have to be established in a test phase of the system for individually for each application.

Referring to the stated requirement from Sect. 4, it can be summarized, that the framework and the exemplary implementation can claim to fulfill the specifications. The described behavior measurement procedure directly measures significant behavior in a useful dimension and works on data from real life scenarios.

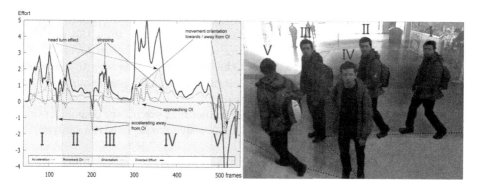

Fig. 6. Directed Effort Scores plotted over time with corresponding behavior illustration. The scene is divided into phases (I–V). (I): Person walking parallel to display with head turned towards the screen. (II) and (III) Person stopping to watch, movement direction still parallel and head turned. (IV) Person approaching the screen changing direction assuming a close and comfortable position with head and shoulders oriented in the same direction. (V) Turning and leaving the scene. The dotted curves show the result for the single components of Directed Effort which are aggregated to an overall score of Directed Effort (solid line). Positive amplitudes express positive contributions, negative amplitudes indicate activities which are directed away from the display.

6   Results

To evaluate the framework functionality, plotting DE scores over time provides useful information. It results in effort curves which are useful to present the applicability and the potential of our effort-based behavior analysis approach. The resulting curves succeed in adequately describing behavior and signal changes of behavior via strong signal peaks. In Fig. 6, the effort curves have been plotted for the single DE parameters acceleration, moving direction, and shoulder and head orientation which contribute to the overall Directed Effort curve, using an example from a database which was gathered during an installation at a public event. This sample has been divided into five sections which mark different behavioral segments.

As can be observed, the calculated DE curve gives a suitable expression of invested physical effort and enables detection and interpretation of behavioral changes. The beginning of each of the sections which indicate different kinds of activities is marked with a strong peak in the DE curve, indicating a high effort level and a substantial change in behavior as demanded in our theoretical approach. The height and width of the peak represent an indicator for the strength of the behavior modification and the algebraic sign clearly separates contributive from detrimental actions. Smaller behavioral changes like the deceleration in Sects. 2 and 3 result in a lower peaks than changes which include strong deviations in more than one of the single parameters, as in Sects. 4 and 5. In the latter sections, the person not only alters movement speed, but as well the movement direction and body orientation resulting in higher DE scores.

The noise-like patterns which occur throughout the sample are mainly caused by oscillations in the acceleration parameter, which derive from the gait frequency and the slightly strolling walking style of the subject. Overall, DE curves show promising stability and at the same time reactivity to behavior modifications and seem to adequately describe the qualitative commitment of people towards objects like public displays.

To demonstrate the functionality of the framework, exemplary demonstration videos have been uploaded at http://www.pervasive.jku.at/behavioranalysis/.

7   Conclusion and Outlook

In this paper, we have presented an approach towards a higher level interpretative description of behavior to express engagement and commitment of via detection of behavior changes. Such an approach can never claim to be able to predict the exact focus of attention of a person but can only try to provide a model which approximates reality through iterative refinement. The more we accomplish a detailed description of behavior and context, the better we will perform in interpreting human behavior. Yet, the proposed methods may provide a first step towards a behavior-based attention estimation.

References

1. Bitgood, S.: Not another step! economy of movement and pedestrian choice point behavior in shopping malls. Environ. Behav. **38**(3), 394–405 (2006). http://eab.sagepub.com/cgi/doi/10.1177/0013916505280081
2. Blank, M., Gorelick, L., Shechtman, E., Irani, M., Basri, R.: Actions as space-time shapes. In: 2005 Tenth IEEE International Conference on Computer Vision, ICCV 2005, vol. 2, pp. 1395–1402 (2005)
3. Bobick, A., Davis, J.: The recognition of human movement using temporal templates. IEEE Trans. Pattern Anal. Mach. Intell. **23**(3), 257–267 (2001)
4. Bongers, K.C., Dijksterhuis, A., Spears, R.: Self-esteem regulation after success and failure to attain unconsciously activated goals. J. Exp. Soc. Psychol. **45**(3), 468–477 (2009). http://www.sciencedirect.com/science/article/pii/S0022103109000031
5. Candamo, J., Shreve, M., Goldgof, D., Sapper, D., Kasturi, R.: Understanding transit scenes: a survey on human behavior-recognition algorithms. IEEE Trans. Intell. Transp. Syst. **11**(1), 206–224 (2010)
6. Cooper, J.O., Heron, T.E., Heward, W.L.: Applied Behavior Analysis, 2nd edn. Pearson/Merrill-Prentice Hall, Upper Saddle River (2007)
7. Dijksterhuis, A., Aarts, H.: Goals, attention, and (un)consciousness. Ann. Rev. Psychol. **61**(1), 467–490 (2010). http://dx.doi.org/10.1146/annurev.psych. 093008.100445
8. Guevara, J.E., Umemuro, H.: Unobtrusive estimation of psychological states based on human movement observation. e-Minds **2**(6), 39–60 (2010)
9. Hietanen, J.: Social attention orienting integrates visual information from head and body orientation. Psychol. Res. **66**(3), 174–179 (2002)
10. Hoffman, J.E., Subramaniam, B.: The role of visual attention in saccadic eye movements. Percept. Psychophys. **57**(6), 787–795 (1995)

11. Hunt, A.R., Kingstone, A.: Covert and overt voluntary attention: linked or independent? Brain research. Cogn. Brain Res. **18**(1), 102–105 (2003)
12. Ji, X., Liu, H.: Advances in view-invariant human motion analysis: a review. IEEE Trans. Syst. Man Cybern. Part C Appl. Rev. **40**(1), 13–24 (2010)
13. Kahneman, D.: Attention and Effort. Prentice-Hall, Englewood Cliffs (1973)
14. Knudsen, E.I.: Fundamental components of attention. Ann. Rev. Neurosci. **30**(1), 57–78 (2007). http://www.ncbi.nlm.nih.gov/pubmed/17417935
15. Moore, T., Fallah, M.: Control of eye movements and spatial attention. Proc. Natl. Acad. Sci. U.S.A **98**(3), 1273–1276 (2001)
16. Müller, H.J., Rabbitt, P.M.: Reflexive and voluntary orienting of visual attention: time course of activation and resistance to interruption. J. Exp. Psychol. Hum. Percept. Performance **15**(2), 315–330 (1989)
17. Perry, R.J.: The neurology of saccades and covert shifts in spatial attention: an event-related fMRI study. Brain **123**(11), 2273–2288 (2000)
18. Peursum, P., Venkatesh, S., West, G.: Tracking-as-recognition for articulated full-body human motion analysis. In: 2007 IEEE Conference on Computer Vision and Pattern Recognition, CVPR '07, pp. 1–8 (2007)
19. Posner, M.I.: Orienting of attention. Q. J. Exp. Psychol. **32**(1), 3–25 (1980)
20. Rizzolatti, G., Riggio, L., Dascola, I., Umiltá, C.: Reorienting attention across the horizontal and vertical meridians: evidence in favor of a premotor theory of attention. Neuropsychologia **25**(1A), 31–40 (1987)
21. Shi, Y., Bobick, A., Essa, I.: Learning temporal sequence model from partially labeled data. In: 2006 IEEE Computer Society Conference on Computer Vision and Pattern Recognition, vol. 2, pp. 1631–1638 (2006)
22. Smith, K.C., Ba, S.O., Odobez, J.M., Gatica-Perez, D.: Tracking attention for multiple people: wandering visual focus of attention estimation. Idiap-RR Idiap-RR-40-2006, IDIAP (2006, submitted for publication)
23. Wickens, C.D., McCarley, J.S.: Applied Attention Theory. CRC Press, Boca Raton (2008). http://www.worldcat.org/oclc/156994621
24. Yakiyama, Y., Thepvilojanapong, N., Iwai, M., Mihirogi, O., Umeda, K., Tobe, Y.: Observing real-world attention by a laser scanner. IPSJ Online Trans. **2**, 93–106 (2009)

Author Index